Con

CW01429326

General preface to the series

Two people having the same operation can have quite different experiences, but one feeling that is common to many is that things might have been easier if they had had a better idea of what to expect. Some people are reluctant to ask questions, and many forget what they are told, sometimes because they are anxious, and sometimes because they do not really understand the explanations they are given.

In most medical centres in Britain today, the emphasis is more on patient involvement than at any time in the past. It is now generally accepted that it is important for people to understand what their treatment entails, both in terms of reducing their stress and thus aiding their recovery, and of making their care more straightforward for the medical staff involved.

The books in this series have been written with the aim of giving people comprehensive information about each of the medical conditions covered, about the treatment they are likely to be offered, and about what may happen during their post-operative recovery period. Armed with this knowledge, you should have the confidence to question, and to take part in the decisions made.

Going in to hospital for the first time can be a daunting experience, and therefore the books describe the procedures involved, and identify and explain the roles of the hospital staff with whom you are likely to come into contact.

Anaesthesia is explained in general terms, and the options

available for a particular operation are described in each book.

There may be complications following any operation – usually minor but none the less worrying for the person involved – and the common ones are described and explained. Now that less time is spent in hospital following most non-emergency operations, knowing what to expect in the days following surgery, and what to do if a complication does arise, is more important than ever before.

Where relevant, the books include a section of exercises and advice to help you to get back to normal and to deal with the everyday activities which can be difficult or painful in the first few days after an operation.

Doctors and nurses, like members of any profession, use a jargon, and they often forget that many of the terms that are familiar to them are not part of everyday language for most of us. Care has been taken to make the books easily understandable by everyone, and each book has a list of simple explanations of the medical terms you may come across.

Most doctors and nurses are more than willing to explain and to discuss problems with patients, but they often assume that if you do not ask questions, you either do not want to know or you know already. Questions and answers are given in every book to help you to draw up your own list to take with you when you see your family doctor or consultant.

Each book also has a section of case histories of people who have experienced the particular operation themselves. These are included to give you an idea of the problems which can arise, problems which may sometimes seem relatively trivial to others but which can be distressing to those directly concerned.

Although the majority of people are satisfied with the medical care they receive, things can go wrong. If you do feel you need to make a complaint about something that happened, or did not happen, during your treatment, each book has a section which deals in detail with how to go about this.

It was the intention in writing these books to help to take some of the worry out of having an operation. It is not knowing what to expect, and the feeling of being involved in some process over which we have no control, and which we do not fully understand, that makes us anxious. The books in the series *Your Operation* should help to remove some of that anxiety and make you feel less like a car being serviced, and more like part of the team of people who are working together to cure your medical problem and put you back on the road to health.

You may not know *all* there is to know about a particular condition when you have read the book related to it, but you will know more than enough to prepare yourself for your operation. You may decide you do not want to go ahead with surgery. Although this is not the authors' intention, they will be happy that you have been given enough information to feel confident to make your own decision, and to take an active part in your own care. After all, it is *your* operation.

Jane Smith
Bristol, 1996

Preface

Our hip joints can function more or less normally for 70 years or more, despite the considerable stress they are subjected to during our lives. But, when problems do arise, the pain and immobility caused by a damaged or diseased hip joint can have a devastating effect on a person's quality of life.

Although significant improvements have been made in hip replacement surgery – both in terms of surgical techniques and of the design and materials used in the manufacture of artificial components – replacement hip joints still only have an expected lifespan of about 15 to 20 years. Revision surgery may therefore be necessary at some time to remove the components which have been inserted and replace them with new ones. It is more likely to be required during the lifetime of anyone who is relatively young when they have their first hip replacement, and the pre-operative assessment necessary for all patients is even more important for this particular group.

This book deals with total and partial hip replacement (hemiarthroplasty), both of which constitute major surgery, explaining what is involved in the two operations and how to look after your new hip. It should also be useful reading for anyone caring for a relative or friend following any type of hip replacement surgery.

Jane Smith
Ian D. Learmonth
Bristol, 1996

Acknowledgements

We are extremely grateful to all the people who gave so generously of their time and knowledge to help in the writing of this book. Particular thanks are due to Ward Sister Thelma Richards, and to Lesley Roper, Superintendent Physiotherapist, Michelle Taplin, Orthopaedic Physiotherapist, and Meg Birch, Occupational Therapy Services Manager – all at the Avon Orthopaedic Centre, Southmead Hospital, Bristol. We are also grateful to Maureen Lee, Research Assistant, University of Bristol.

Special thanks go to the men and women who related their own experiences for the section of case histories.

CHAPTER 1

Introduction

Approximately one million hip replacement operations are done each year worldwide: some 40 000 of them in the UK and 250 000 in the USA. Although most people who undergo this type of surgery are over the age of 65, about a quarter are younger than 55. Damage to the hip joint can result from various disorders, but the most common cause is arthritis.

Surgery to replace all or part of a diseased hip joint can have a dramatic effect on the lifestyle of someone suffering severe pain and disability, but it is a major operation which should not be undertaken lightly. Your family doctor or consultant will be able to advise you of the likely benefits of surgery in your particular case, but the final decision to go ahead is yours, and before making it you should be sure that your expectations about its outcome are realistic and that you understand what is involved. It is hoped that this book will provide enough information to help you make an informed decision.

There are several terms you may come across in any discussion of hip replacement surgery, and it is useful to know what they mean. **Arthropathy** is any disease which affects a joint. **Arthroplasty** is an operation to alleviate pain and restore function of a joint by excision or by replacing it with artificial components, known as **prostheses**. There are several different types of arthroplasty. The two operations dealt with in this book are **total hip replacement (THR)**, which involves complete replacement of the head of the thigh bone and the lining of the joint socket on the pelvis, and **hemi-arthroplasty**, which involves replacement of one half of the hip joint, normally the head of the thigh bone.

Other types of hip surgery include **osteotomy** and **interpositional arthroplasty**. Osteotomy involves cutting through the femur to change its alignment and alter the direction of the force exerted across the joint, thus transferring the stress of walking away from a diseased area of the bone to another, healthy part. Interpositional arthroplasty may be performed to interpose a material between the joint surfaces or bone ends to keep them apart.

To understand what happens when the hip joint becomes diseased or damaged, it is helpful to know something of its anatomy and function.

THE HIP JOINT

The hip itself is made up of two large bones, joined in front at the **symphysis pubis** and forming the **sacrum** at the rear. Each of the two hip bones is made up of three parts – the **ilium**, **ischium** and **pubis** – which fuse during childhood. Together, the two hip bones form the **pelvis**, which protects the internal pelvic organs.

The thigh bone, known as the **femur**, is the longest bone in the body. Its head is curved and fits into a cup-shaped cavity (the **acetabulum**) on the outer side of the hip bone, forming a **ball-and-socket joint**. There are also two bony processes on the upper part of the femur, called **trochanters**, to which various muscles are attached.

The surface of the head of the femur (the ball) and the socket formed by the acetabulum are covered by specialised gristle-like tissue called **articular cartilage**. Attached to the rim of the articular cartilage is a capsule of strong fibrous tissue enclosing the **joint cavity**. Thickened strands of the capsule form **ligaments** which support the joint.

The joint cavity is lined by a membrane called the **synovium**, the cells of which secrete an oily **synovial fluid** to lubricate the articulating surfaces of the joint and allow smooth movement of

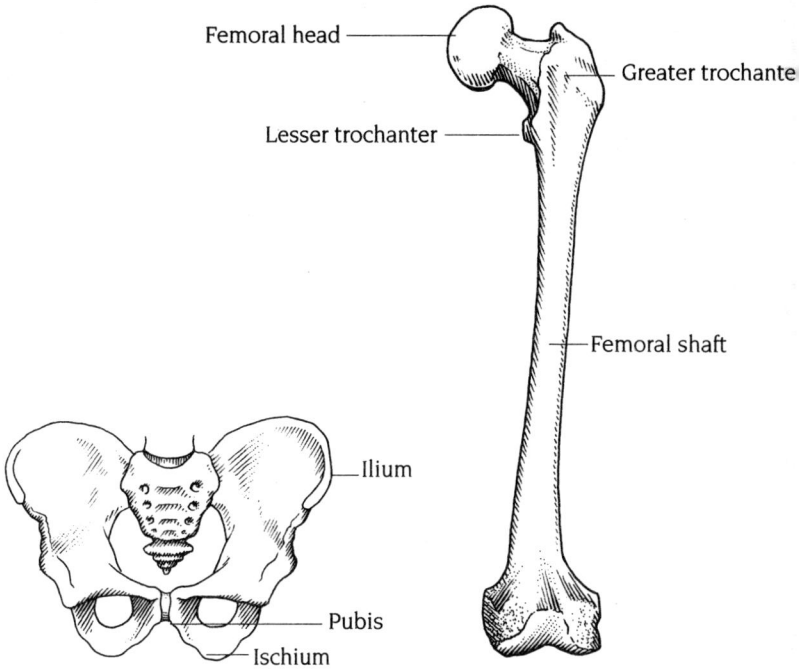

Femoral head

Greater trochante

Lesser trochanter

Femoral shaft

Ilium

Pubis

Ischium

The pelvis.

The femur.

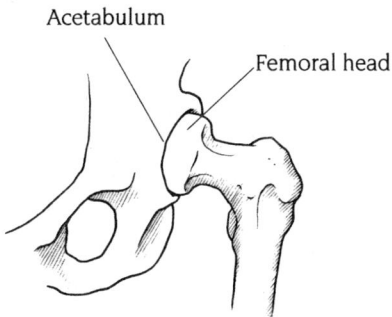

Acetabulum

Femoral head

The bones of the hip joint. This diagram shows how the ball-shaped head of the thigh bone fits into the socket in the pelvis.

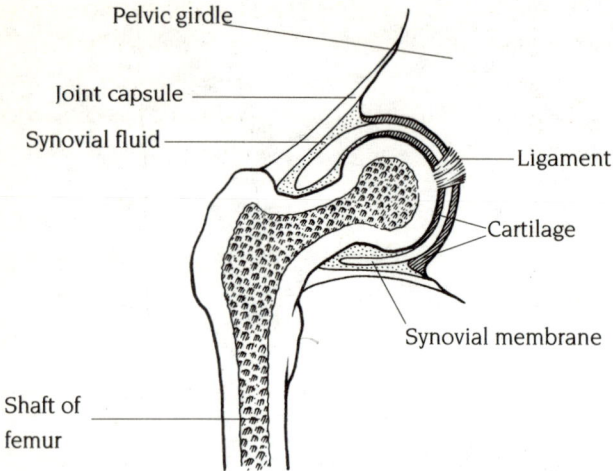

A typical ball-and-socket joint, such as that of the hip.

the ball within the socket. The joint also has a network of blood vessels, lymph vessels and nerves.

Movement of the hip joint

The hip joint can undertake a range of movements in different planes, some or all of which may be lost following hip disease of long standing. The movements can be grouped into pairs of opposite actions as follows. **Flexion** is bending of the joint forwards; **extension** is bending it backwards. **Internal rotation** is turning the joint inwards; **external rotation** is turning it outwards. **Abduction** is raising the leg to the side; **adduction** is crossing one leg over the other.

When movement in the joint is lost, the soft tissues and muscles around it shorten, leading to **contracture**. The most common problem following disease of the hip joint is **flexion contracture**: the joint can bend forward to a variable degree but cannot be fully straightened. Flexion contracture may lead to difficulty tying your shoelaces, cutting your toenails etc. As loss of movement occurs, more strain is placed on the spine and knee, often causing back pain. Eventually the hip develops flexion, adduction and external rotation deformities, at which point various movements such as getting in and out of a car become difficult.

There are several sets of muscles around the hip joint, the most important being the three **gluteal** muscles responsible for abduction and extension. The **psoas** muscle controls flexion and internal rotation; and the **gemelli** and **quadratus femoris** muscles control external rotation. There are also **adductor** muscles, a **rectus femoris**, **pectineus**, **iliacus**, and **tensor fascia lata**.

Biomechanics of the hip joint

During all the activities of daily life, considerable force is exerted at the articular surfaces of the hip joint, both vertically and horizontally. A force approximately equal to three to four times the weight of your body is exerted during walking. This force may increase tenfold during running or when taking part in vigorous sporting activities. Thus the hip joint of a man weighing 80 kg must absorb a force of up to 800 kg when, for example, he is playing squash. Therefore, the physical demands made on the hip joint over the years are enormous and the fact that it can normally continue to function for so long with little sign of wear constitutes an unparalleled feat of engineering design.

CAUSES OF PROBLEMS WITH THE HIP JOINT

There are several problems and diseases which can affect the hip joint (as well as other joints in the body), causing damage to the bones and other tissues and eventually pain and reduced mobility. The more severe the pain and disability you have suffered before surgery, the more dramatic its effects are likely to be. Operations are also sometimes done to correct deformity of the hip joint caused by disease or shortening of the muscles around it. However, deformity alone is not generally sufficient reason for surgery, except when it makes walking difficult and/or is accompanied by pain.

Pain

Damage to the hip joint can often result in pain deep in the groin, in the buttock or in the thigh. Pain may also sometimes be *referred* from the hip to other parts of the body, such as the knee or lower in the leg. Occasionally it may be referred *to* the hip joint from the spine or pelvis, from a hernia or even a prostate problem in men or an ovarian cyst in women. In older people with generalised arthritis, pain often co-exists in both the hip and the back. It is therefore important to identify the exact cause of a painful or immobile hip joint whenever possible. Pain which is referred to the hip is sometimes diagnosed by injecting a drug into the hip to anaesthetise it for a few hours. If the same pain is still felt in the region of the anaesthetised hip, it is likely to be referred pain and the cause is unlikely to be the hip itself. However, if the pain around the hip is abolished by the injection into the joint, it is probable that the hip is the main problem.

If the hip joint is completely destroyed by disease, the pain felt in it may decrease, although the strain normally taken up by the hip during walking etc. may then be transferred to other joints such as those of the knee and spine. In these cases, despite the lack of pain, a hip replacement operation may be done to protect the other joints from further damage.

Osteoarthritis

Osteoarthritis is the most common form of chronic joint disease. It results from destruction and degeneration of the cartilage at the articular surfaces of joints and may cause progressive joint pain and stiffness. The hip and knee are most commonly affected, particularly in the elderly.

There are various types of osteoarthritis, the causes of which are not always known. It may be associated with gout, infection or injury of a joint, or may occur as a result of the death (**necrosis**) of areas of bone due to alcoholism or to the long-term use of steroids or anti-inflammatory drugs. It can also develop (most commonly in the knee) in people with haemophilia: repeated bleeding into the joint results in swelling and inflammation, with subsequent destruction of the articular cartilage.

In younger people, osteoarthritis may be the result of congenital dislocation of a joint (i.e. dislocation which has been present from birth), damage caused by fracture, or previous inflammation. Any abnormality which puts an unusual stress on the joint can also predispose to this disease, as can excessive use – or misuse – of the joint, for example due to strenuous physical activity.

In the early stages of osteoarthritis, the cartilage at the ends of the bones alters in structure and may begin to flake. Once the cartilage is lost, the surface of the bone beneath becomes exposed. By this time, the bone is likely to be more dense than normal and its exposed surface may become grooved. The head of the femur flattens into a mushroom shape and patches of bone may be replaced by pockets of degenerate fibrous tissue. Small growths of cartilage, known as **osteophytes**, may form at the joint margins and become covered in bony material (**ossified**), possibly restricting movement of the joint.

Although the synovium is normal in the early stages of osteoarthritis, it gradually changes in character as the joint surface disintegrates, leading to inflammation known as **synovitis**. Excessive synovial fluid may then escape into the joint cavity.

Sometimes osteoarthritis can progress rapidly while remaining painless. Because of the lack of pain, the joint continues to be used until the cartilage is destroyed and the ends of the bone are damaged. If the condition does cause pain, it may be worse in damp, cold weather and in people who are overweight and whose weight-bearing hip joints are therefore under abnormal stress. In the early stages, pain may be relieved by simple painkillers such as paracetamol. Occasionally, injections of non-steroidal anti-inflammatory drugs may be given if the pain continues, although the inaccessibility of the hip joint makes this option uncommon.

The management of osteoarthritis may include the use of aids such as canes or crutches to assist mobility, weight reduction by modifying the diet when necessary, stopping any inappropriate exercise which may be exacerbating the condition, physiotherapy to restore the strength in the muscles and the mobility of the joints as well as to help relieve pain, and drug therapy to reduce pain and inflammation.

Rheumatoid arthritis

Rheumatoid arthritis is a disease of the connective tissues which involves inflammation of several joints. It often first becomes apparent between the ages of 25 and 55, although it can affect older and younger people. It is more common in women and can cause severe crippling. The affected joints become swollen and tender, due both to synovitis and to the escape of synovial fluid into the joint cavity. The bones eventually become demineralised and the muscles weak and atrophied. Although the disease often burns itself out in time, any damaged joints will continue to disintegrate.

Osteoporosis

Osteoporosis is a reduction in the density of bone which can occur as a result of decreased bone formation and/or increased bone resorption. As the bone tissue is lost, the bones become brittle and tend to fracture as a result of minor injury. Osteoporosis may also result in collapse of the head of the

INTRODUCTION

femur and subsequent hip-joint problems. Its precise cause is unknown, but it is an exaggeration of the natural process which occurs with age and which begins in men and women in their thirties. It can be localised or diffuse and may, for example, follow atrophy of the bones due to immobilisation or paralysis. The condition is common in post-menopausal women, suggesting an association in some cases with lack of the hormone oestrogen, production of which decreases after the menopause or following removal of the ovaries. Hormone replacement therapy (HRT) is therefore often used to treat osteoporosis.

Fractures

Hip-joint fractures are associated with osteoporosis and are relatively common in elderly people, although they can occur at any age.

A common site of fracture is across the neck of the femur. The blood supply to the bone above the fracture may be interrupted and the head of the femur may then die, resulting in secondary deformity and subsequent arthritis. Hemi-arthroplasty (see p.1) may be the treatment of choice for this type of fracture.

A BRIEF HISTORY OF JOINT REPLACEMENT

The first attempts at surgery to replace damaged hip joints were made as long ago as the early 1800s. Although the techniques and materials have improved since those early pioneering days, in many cases the operations done today are refined versions of the original ones.

Osteotomy for example (see p.2) was first performed in the USA in 1826 and is still done successfully today. Interpositional arthroplasty (see p.2) has also been practised since the last century. Many implant materials have been used, with variable success, including muscle, silver, rubber, glass, Pyrex, wax, pig's

9

bladder, gold foil and a cobalt/chrome alloy called Vitallium, first used in 1923 and still giving quite satisfactory results more than 70 years later.

In 1822, the first **excision arthroplasty** was done in London. The operation involves cutting away one or both sides of a joint (the head of the femur in operations on the hip joint) to reduce pain and preserve mobility. Although it had some success at the time and was widely practised before the introduction of total hip replacement, it is rarely done today.

Replacement hemi-arthroplasty was first performed in 1919, replacing the head of the femur with a rubber prosthesis. In 1927, rubber was superseded by ivory and in 1940 by metal. A few years later, acrylic was thought to be a superior material for this operation, but it was found to wear badly and eventually to fracture. However, the surgical technique was refined and evolved into the operation done today.

Total hip replacement was first attempted in Germany in 1891 with an ivory ball-and-socket joint fixed to the bone with nickel-plated screws. In England in 1938, stainless steel prostheses were fixed with screws and bolts, but the results were unsatisfactory.

Despite the frequent disappointments, prosthesis development continued, and by the 1950s good long-term results were starting to be achieved with cement and metal components. At this time, a clinician called John Charnley dominated the field of total hip replacement surgery. His work led to the development of implant materials which produced little friction and were self-lubricating and of components which could be fixed to living bone by a quick-setting acrylic cement. Obtaining unsatisfactory results with prostheses made of Teflon – which wore badly and produced particles which gave rise to serious foreign body reactions – Charnley then tried a high molecular weight polyethylene (HMWP) which has been refined and is still in use today.

Implant fixation and prosthetic materials continue to evolve as technology and surgical techniques improve (see Chapter 3).

CHAPTER 2

Tests and decisions

Most people considering a hip replacement operation will have had pain and possibly increasing mobility problems for some time. If treatment with drugs and physiotherapy has gradually become less effective, your doctor may suggest the possibility of surgery and may refer you to an **orthopaedic consultant** for examination and assessment. An orthopaedic consultant is a doctor who specialises in abnormalities, diseases and injuries of the locomotor system, i.e. all parts of the body involved in locomotion.

VISITING A CONSULTANT

Your family doctor will write to an orthopaedic consultant from whom you should receive a letter giving the date and time of your appointment and any other relevant information. Although your appointment will be at a particular consultant's clinic, you may be seen by another doctor in the consultant's 'firm' rather than by the consultant him or herself. During your out-patient appointment, a hospital doctor will take details of your medical history and may also question you about the health and causes of death of your near relatives. Movement in your hip joint will be assessed, together with your ability to walk and any associated limp. You will be asked about the extent to which your disability interferes with your daily activities, such as going up and down stairs, putting on your stockings or socks etc., and about the degree and pattern of your pain and anything which makes it worse or better. X-rays will probably be taken of both your hip joints to help diagnose the cause of your problem and to assess the existing damage.

It is important that a clear picture is built up of your general state of health and pattern of daily life so that a decision can be made about whether surgery is the right option for you. The doctor will also need to be satisfied that the risks of surgery and anaesthesia will not be increased by complications caused by any other illness or disability you may have. However, it is possible to undergo hip arthroplasty even if you do have other medical problems or are elderly. If necessary, special tests may be arranged and an appointment may be made for you to be examined by a specialist in another branch of medicine – such as a heart specialist – to obtain an opinion about whether you are fit for surgery.

Obesity

Obesity adds to the risk of general anaesthesia and can make surgery more difficult. Excess weight can also put additional strain on a replacement hip joint, possibly shortening its lifespan. Some surgeons are therefore reluctant to carry out non-emergency operations on obese patients as they consider the risks to be too great. However, starting a long, strict diet before your operation may be inadvisable and your weight will be assessed and you will be given any necessary guidance by the hospital doctor.

MAKING A DECISION

There are several factors which need to be considered before a decision can be made to go ahead with surgery. As has already been mentioned, your doctor can advise you about the likely effects of surgery in your particular case, but the final decision must be made by you, bearing in mind your lifestyle, whether the pain you are suffering could be controlled by other means, and whether your expectations are realistic in terms of what you hope can be achieved by an operation. The decision about whether or not to opt for surgery is therefore very patient specific and will be influenced by the demands you place on your hip: active people are likely to consider hip replacement sooner than people who are relatively sedentary.

The following factors will have to be taken into account to assess whether surgery is the most appropriate treatment for you.

* _Your age._ If you are elderly, will hip replacement more or less guarantee a lifetime free of pain and be unlikely to need revision? (Replacement hips have a finite life, which can be reduced by vigorous physical activity). If you are younger and hope to lead a very active life, would it be better to postpone an operation to await further advances in technology which might enable you to do so?

* _The cause of your hip problem._

* _The quality of your bone and muscle._ As the components of a replacement hip have to be inserted into existing bone, an operation may not be feasible if the quality of your bones is generally poor.

* _Your general physical condition._ For example, do you have other arthritic joints which will continue to restrict your daily life, or a serious medical condition which might increase the risks of surgery and anaesthesia?

* _Alternatives to total hip replacement._ Would the advantages of total hip replacement far outweigh those of other types of surgery or of non-surgical treatments?

* _Realistic expectations._ Are you likely to deal well with the period of hospitalisation involved, and to be committed to the

rehabilitation process necessary post-operatively? Relatively young people who seek surgery in the hope of continuing to take part in strenuous sporting activities should be aware that it will not realise this ambition for them. For example, you may have to accept the fact that you will have to give up playing squash and perhaps take up a less active sport.

* *Real need*. People who lead very sedentary lives and who perhaps spend much of their time at home may be better advised to consider non-surgical treatment to control any pain caused by a hip problem. Total hip replacement is a major operation which is more appropriate for those wishing to resume a fairly active lifestyle.

Bilateral hip replacement If both your hips are badly affected, it may be necessary to consider replacing both joints in one operation. This option would be indicated, for example, if the pain in both hip joints is so bad that only replacing one would severely restrict any attempt at rehabilitation after surgery. Severe deformity may also be an indication for replacing both hips at once as, if only one hip joint is replaced, it could adopt the deformity of the unreplaced one.

However, replacing both hips at the same time involves a much bigger operation and would not be considered for anyone who is frail or has contraindications such as heart or chest problems.

Once the doctor has decided that an operation is appropriate and has discussed all the relevant factors with you, you may want to ask for time to think about it and to talk it over with your family or friends before you make a final decision. Do make sure to ask any questions you may have and do not be afraid to ask for an explanation of anything which is not clear to you.

TESTS AND EXAMINATIONS

If you decide to have surgery and are put on a waiting list, there are several tests which may need to be done. In most cases, these tests can be carried out at a **pre-operative assessment clinic** (see p.27) a few weeks or days before you enter hospital to allow time for the results to be obtained before your operation. If the tests reveal any infection or abnormality, your operation may have to be postponed while it is treated (see p.28).

You are likely to have the pre-operative tests described below, and may also have others specifically related to any pre-existing condition, such as a liver function test if you are known to have liver disease or damage.

* X-*rays*. A chest X-ray will be done to detect any respiratory condition which could complicate the use of a general anaesthetic or which will need to be treated before or after your operation.

    As it may be several months since an X-ray was taken of your hip at your out-patients' appointment, another may be done to detect any change in the hip joint which may have occurred in the intervening period.

* An *electrocardiogram*. An electrocardiogram (ECG) will be done to check that your heart is functioning normally and is healthy enough to withstand surgery. If you do have any cardiovascular problems, it may still be possible for your operation to go ahead, but it is important that the surgeon and anaesthetist are aware of them so that any necessary precautions can be taken, both during and after surgery.

    As the heart beats, its muscle produces a wave of electrical energy, the pattern and size of which can be recorded via electrodes taped to the skin. A normal heart produces a distinctive pattern of electrical waves; an abnormal pattern indicates some dysfunction of the heart, such as a poor blood supply, abnormal rhythm or weak heart muscle.

During the test, electrodes will be attached to your wrists and ankles and then to the skin over your chest. The electrocardiogram is simple and straightforward, but it is important that you lie as still as possible during the few minutes it takes to do it so that electrical impulses generated by the movement of other muscles do not mask those from the heart. (Electrodes from a similar ECG monitor will also be attached to your chest throughout your operation to make sure your heart rhythm remains normal.)

*   *Blood tests*. A sample of your blood will be taken to measure its haemoglobin level. Oxygen is essential for the health and repair of the tissues of the body and for wound healing, and it is transported in the blood attached to haemoglobin. Blood will inevitably be lost during surgery, and if your level of haemoglobin is already low, it will fall even further. Therefore, if your haemoglobin level is found to be substantially below normal or you are anaemic, you may be prescribed a course of iron tablets to correct the problem before your operation.

    Some 30 per cent of people having total hip replacement surgery will require a blood transfusion, and it is therefore also important that your blood is cross-matched so that blood of the correct group can be made available in case you need it.

*   *Urinalysis*. Urinary tract infection can give rise to postoperative infection elsewhere (with potentially serious consequences if it spreads to your hip). As urinary tract infections can be present without causing any symptoms, a sample of your urine will be analysed to detect the presence of infective organisms. If necessary, you will be given antibiotics to clear up any infection before your operation.

At some stage before your operation, possibly at a pre-operative assessment appointment, you will be asked about any drugs you are taking, about your medical history, any infection you may have, any past problems with bleeding, and if you have ever suffered any ill-effects from an anaesthetic. You will be given a thorough physical examination, including an examination of the range of movement in your affected hip joint, and may also undergo one or both of the following procedures.

IMAGING TECHNIQUES

There are various imaging techniques which can be used to obtain a picture of the hip joint and to enable the surgeon to select the most appropriate joint implant and surgical procedure for you.

Computed tomography

Computed tomography (CT) is a method of producing a series of images of the body which are interpreted by a computer. You will be asked to lie on a table which will be passed through a large hoop-shaped scanner. The various images produced by the scanner will be assembled by a computer and presented as X-ray pictures of cross-sectional slices through your body.

Magnetic resonance imaging

Magnetic resonance imaging (MRI) produces images without the use of X-rays. It allows good depiction of the body's soft tissues and of any abnormalities within the bone marrow.

Like computed tomography, magnetic resonance imaging is a form of scan, providing information which is interpreted by a computer. The scanner in this case is a large, high-powered magnet contained within a scanning tunnel. Again, you will be asked to lie on a table which will pass through a tunnel as the series of scans is taken.

As the procedure involves the use of a magnet, you must not take anything metal into the scanning tunnel, and it is unsuitable, for example, for anyone with a cardiac pacemaker. Some people find the tunnel claustrophobic and may be sedated before having this scan.

CHAPTER 3

Prostheses

Once a decision has been made to go ahead with surgery, the surgeon will have to decide on the best materials and type of prosthesis to use in your particular case. This selection will depend on factors such as your age and normal level of activity as well as on the degree of damage and deterioration of the bones of your hip joint. Although a replacement hip joint may continue to function successfully for 15 years or more, it will not last for ever. Careful consideration is therefore necessary before replacing the hip of someone in their forties or fifties, who is likely to require revision surgery at some time in the future (see Chapter 11). In this instance, a cementless prosthesis which will preserve bone stock may be most appropriate.

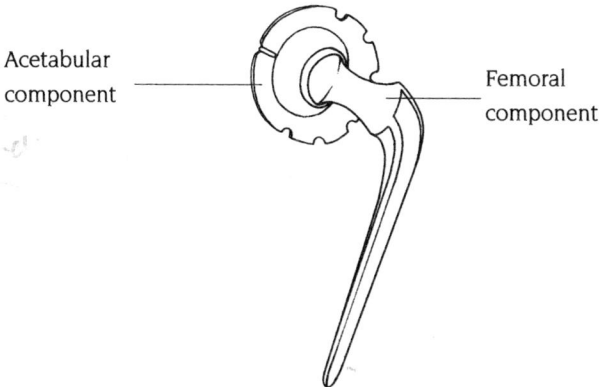

Acetabular component

Femoral component

Charnley prostheses. These are examples of components often used to replace the head of the femur and the lining of the acetabulum in the pelvic bone.

The ultimate aim of total hip replacement is to insert a prosthesis (component) into the existing bone – with either cemented or cementless fixation – which will last indefinitely without needing to be replaced. To date, no such perfect prosthesis has been developed and thus the already wide array of options is constantly being modified and added to. For example, the use of a cementless acetabular prosthesis and a cement-fixed femoral prosthesis – so-called **hybrid replacement** – seems to give good results, although no information is yet available concerning its success in the longer term.

THE FEMORAL COMPONENT

The femoral component is the prosthesis which replaces the head of the femur. Apart from a ball-shaped *head*, the prosthesis usually also has a *stem* which is inserted into the shaft of the femur itself; a *neck* between the head and the stem; and a *shoulder* at the junction between the neck and the stem. There may also be a *collar* which rests on the top of the inner aspect of the femur. The femoral component may be made of any one of a variety of metals (see p.22).

THE ACETABULAR COMPONENT

The acetabular component comprises a *cup* or *socket* which rests on the existing acetabular bone. The majority of acetabular components are made of a lightweight, strong, organic compound called a **polymer** which, for cementless components, may be metal backed.

MATERIALS

Whether or not a hip replacement is successful depends to a large extent on the amount of friction between the articulating surfaces of the femoral head and acetabular cup. Friction at

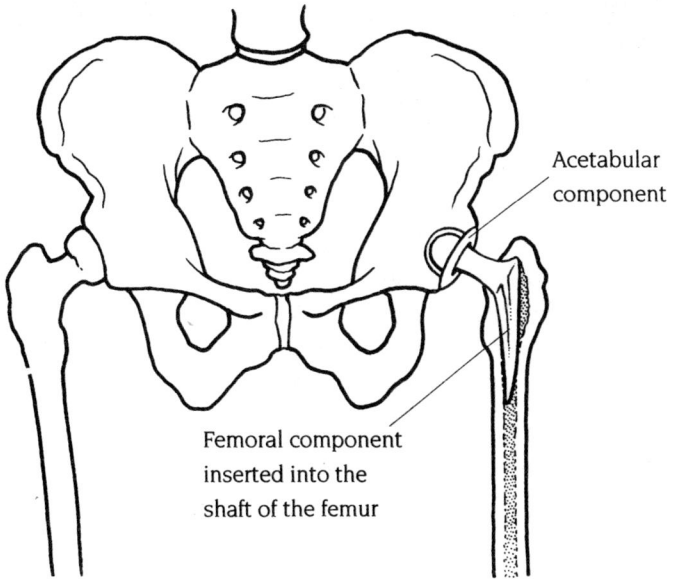

Total hip replacement. This diagram shows a femoral and an acetabular component inserted to replace the bones of the hip joint.

this point leads to the production of **wear debris** as small particles are rubbed off. The wear debris causes inflammation which in turn causes the bone itself to become broken down and absorbed – a process known as **osteolysis**. This can result in loosening of the components and failure of the joint. Many different combinations of materials have therefore been tried over the years in an attempt to overcome this problem. Whereas metal-on-plastic articulations are fine for the majority of people, metal-on-metal designs currently seem to hold the best promise of success for younger, more active patients. Although this discovery may seem somewhat ironic, as it apparently brings hip replacement surgery back to where it started, it is now thought that the failure of many early metal-on-metal joints was due to their engineering design rather than to the materials used.

The following is a very brief review of some of the materials now employed in hip replacement surgery.

Metals

* *Titanium* and *titanium alloys* are strong, light metals which are very biocompatible, i.e. they allow bone to grow relatively easily onto their surface. However, they are scratch and notch sensitive, the latter property sometimes leading to unexpected failure of the implant.

* *Cobalt chrome* is a very strong alloy which has a high resistance to wear and to corrosion.

* *Stainless steel* was used in the original Charnley prosthesis but tended to fracture. A new super steel has now been developed which is much stronger.

Polyethylene

Polyethylene comprises a family of plastics with similar chemical composition but different structures and thus different mechanical and wear properties. The polyethylene used to make acetabular cups has very good wear properties.

Ceramic

Ceramic materials such as zirconium oxide, aluminium oxide and titanium oxide are being used increasingly for one articulating surface of replacement hip joints (often the head of the femur), particularly in young, active people. Ceramic components are brittle but hard, do not scratch easily, are durable and have low friction.

The fixing material

Cement is often used to fix prostheses in place, although some are designed to be inserted without it. The choice depends in part on the preferred practice of your particular surgeon and on factors such as the condition of your existing bone, your age and your activity profile.

Cement

Bone cement is formed by mixing a powder polymer with a liquid monomer. It is a brittle material which degrades with time. It is also porous and can crack if pockets of air are left in it, a problem which may be overcome by mixing it in a vacuum or centrifuging it before use.

During total hip replacement, the acetabulum and femur are prepared and filled with cement into which the prosthesis is inserted. The cement acts as a grout rather than a glue, and once it has set, it fills the gap around the prosthesis and holds it in place. Sometimes a femoral component is precoated with the fixing material before surgery to improve its bonding properties. A substance called **polymethylmethacrylate** (first used by John Charnley, see p.10) is still the most common fixing material but, while it has given extremely good service, there are some problems associated with its use. For example, if it extrudes through a hole in the bone and into the pelvis, it can cause damage to the soft tissues. It is also difficult to remove if revision surgery is required. However, at present its advantages appear to outweigh any disadvantages it may have.

Cementless fixing

Various cementless prostheses have been developed which are mainly used for younger people. However, they are currently less common in the UK than in other parts of Europe and the USA.

Cementless prostheses should be made of a biocompatible material which will allow an intimate bond to form between the bone and the prosthesis. Early attempts at achieving cementless fixation with a polished cemented stem were unsuccessful, and fixation was enhanced by securing the prosthesis to the shaft of the femur with screws.

Stability can be achieved with a good press-fit prosthesis made of biocompatible material, but many of the current cementless prostheses employ some form of biological fixation. For example, the prosthesis can be coated with tiny cobalt chrome beads, hydroxyapatite or titanium mesh which encourage bone ingrowth, known as **osseo-integration**. Too much or too little stress on the bone may cause bone resorption and predispose to failure of the implant. While the short-term results of biological fixation are encouraging, its long-term performance has yet to be proven.

None of the attempts at cementless fixation has so far been found to be superior to the use of cement, which still remains the best option for hip replacement. However, trials are underway to assess the effect of coating prostheses with various other biologically active materials which have a bone-like structure.

CHAPTER 4

Before your operation

Although you will be offered the loan of various aids to assist you during the period of rehabilitation after your operation, there are aids available which could ease some of your problems *before* surgery. It is therefore worth contacting your local social services department and asking to talk to an occupational therapist (see p.73) about, for example, borrowing a raised toilet seat and blocks to increase the height of your bed and a chair while you are awaiting surgery. If necessary, arrangements may be made for an occupational therapist to visit you at home to advise you about any changes which could be made to help you manage more easily. However, in many areas there is a waiting list for these services, which may be up to one year. An alternative is to contact the *Disabled Living Foundation* (see p.137) for information about any shops in your area where equipment is sold and where you can try out the various aids before deciding to buy any which would be useful to you.

PREPARING YOUR HOME

While you are in hospital, you will probably be told several times, by different medical staff, of the importance of avoiding bending down or raising your operated leg for several weeks after your operation. Your legs and the trunk of your body should never be brought close enough together to make an angle of less than 90 degrees, i.e. an L shape. You may also find it difficult to stretch upwards for a time after your operation. Therefore it is a good idea to rearrange things on shelves and in your fridge and cupboards etc. *before* you go into hospital so that anything you are likely to need will be within easy reach.

Have a good look at your home: it is surprising how may things we get used to which could present dangers when mobility is limited. Loose rugs or mats should be taken up to avoid you slipping on them, and any frayed edges to carpets or other potential hazards in which you could catch your foot or which could trip you up should be dealt with.

If you have an unruly dog or a cat which gets under your feet, try to arrange for it to be cared for elsewhere for the first few weeks after your operation. A fall could cause your new hip to dislocate (see p.94) and at the very least could set back the progress you have already made.

Although you will need someone to shop for you for at least a few days after you are discharged from hospital, it may be a good idea to make sure you have a small stock of essential items before you are admitted.

HOME VISITS BY AN OCCUPATIONAL THERAPIST

In some areas, occupational therapists from hospitals make home visits a couple of weeks or so before people are admitted for hip replacement surgery. The purpose of these visits, where they do occur, is to help identify any potential problem areas within people's homes so that they can be sorted out before they enter hospital, or at least before they are discharged after their operation.

Some common problems are chairs and beds which are too low, which can be raised on special blocks loaned by the hospital (see p.84), and toilets with low seats or positioned too far from a wall or other means of support, for which raised toilet seats and rails can be fitted (see pp.85–6).

The occupational therapist will assess your home with a view to helping you cope as easily as possible after your operation, and will advise you about any minor alterations which could be made. If, for example, you need a handrail by some steps or to help you get in and out of the bath, arrangements can often be made for one to be fitted either before you enter hospital or while you are there if there is someone who can let the fitters in to your house and stay with them while the work is done.

PRE-OPERATIVE ASSESSMENT CLINIC

You may be given an appointment to attend a pre-operative assessment clinic some time before your operation. At many hospitals, tests are done at these clinics so that their results are available, and any necessary treatment can be given, before people are admitted for surgery. At the clinic, a doctor will explain your operation and answer any questions you may have. You should be told about the possible risks associated specifically with hip replacement surgery, such as post-operative dislocation and infection, and with operations in general, such as deep vein thrombosis. Do make sure you understand these risks and that you are quite happy to go ahead with surgery. You may be asked to sign a **consent form** at this time, so it is particularly important that you are aware of what is involved in your operation before you do so.

Consent forms   By signing a consent form you are declaring that your operation has been explained to you and that you understand what it entails, and any risks involved, and have agreed to it taking place. You are also giving your permission for the doctors to take whatever action they feel to be appropriate should some emergency occur during surgery, and for any necessary anaesthetic to be given to you. Do read this form carefully, and ask the doctor to explain anything you do not understand.

Hip replacement is a major operation and a chest X-ray and electrocardiogram will be done at the assessment clinic to detect any underlying respiratory or heart disease which could complicate the use of an anaesthetic. A sample of your urine will also be taken and analysed for the presence of urinary tract infection which could lead to more serious infection after your operation. If you are found to have a urinary infection, you will probably be put on a course of antibiotic tablets for five to seven days, at the end of which you will be told to take a further sample of urine to your family doctor. You should ring your doctor three to five days later (or as advised) to find out the results of your urine test. If the antibiotics have failed to clear the infection, it is best to ring the hospital ward or your consultant's secretary as your operation may have to be postponed for a couple of weeks to allow for further treatment. If this does occur, you will not go back on the general waiting list for surgery; your operation will almost certainly be done within two to four weeks at most.

> **When surgery has to be postponed** It is important that medical staff are aware of *any* infection you may have (for example of your chest or urinary tract), of any underlying disease or condition, or of the presence of a leg ulcer or cut etc., however trivial these problems may seem to you. Although it may be tempting not to mention a minor ailment – particularly if you have waited several months for hip surgery and cannot bear the thought of having it cancelled – it is vital that you do so. Infection can be introduced through even a small cut on the leg, with possibly devastating results if your hip were to become infected and the replacement joint had to be removed). Having to have your operation postponed for a couple of weeks because of an existing infection or other problem would be a small price to pay when compared to the potential risks of going ahead with anaesthesia and surgery if you are less than fit.

An occupational therapist may be present at the assessment clinic to explain the process of rehabilitation after your operation and to discuss any problems you might have in caring for yourself when you are discharged from hospital. Do make sure that you mention any difficulties you could face, however minor they may seem to you. Most problems can be overcome and there are various types of help available, but the more time there is to make arrangements for when you leave hospital, the better.

You should take with you to the pre-operative clinic a note of the heights of your bed, toilet and any chairs you will want to sit on so that appropriate aids can be ordered for you to take home after your operation. Although shorter people are less likely to need to raise the height of their furniture, it is helpful if everyone supplies this information.

If any problems are highlighted during your pre-operative assessment, a medical social worker can be alerted to visit you on the ward while you are in hospital to discuss the assistance which may be available when you are discharged, such as 'meals on wheels' or a home help.

You should also mention if you will have difficulty arranging transport to take you home when you are discharged so that nursing staff are aware that hospital transport will need to be booked for you. However, it is better to ask a friend or relative to collect you from hospital if at all possible – and you will certainly need someone to help you at home for at least the first few days.

CHAPTER 5

Going in to hospital for an operation

Normal practice and procedures vary from hospital to hospital, and from surgeon to surgeon. The details given in this chapter about what is likely to happen when you are admitted to hospital for hip replacement surgery are therefore relatively general.

You will receive a letter from the hospital telling you the date of your operation and any other details you need to know, and may also be sent a leaflet explaining the admission procedures and what to take in with you.

If you have already attended a pre-operative assessment clinic, you are likely to be admitted to hospital on the day before your operation, otherwise you will probably be admitted a day or two before surgery for any necessary tests to be done. Once the results of these tests are known, your operation will be able to go ahead. The stay in hospital after hip replacement surgery may be anything between five days and two weeks. (Day-case surgery is not appropriate for any type of hip replacement operation.)

WHAT TO TAKE IN TO HOSPITAL

As you may be in hospital for up to two weeks, there are a few things you will need to take in with you. The following list may be helpful.

1   *Nightclothes*. You will be given a hospital gown to wear during your operation but will need your own loose-fitting night-

clothes, some slippers and a dressing gown before and after it. For example a nightdress can easily be pulled up over your hips to allow you to use a bedpan and for your wound to be checked post-operatively. Pyjama trousers will be left off altogether in the first few hours after surgery and some men find it more comfortable to wear boxer shorts instead of pyjama trousers throughout their hospital stay.

Slippers which provide good support to your feet are more comfortable and safer than floppy slippers or mules. However, your leg is likely to be swollen after your operation which, together with the additional bulk of anti-embolism stockings (see p.39), may make it impossible to get your feet into tight-fitting or new and unworn slippers.

2   *Clothes*. There is no reason why you should continue to wear your nightclothes once you are up and mobile after your operation. Shoes should provide good support to your feet without being tight, and should be flat or have a low heel. Slip-on shoes are preferable to any with buckles or laces as you will not be able to bend to do these up for some time after your operation. High-heeled shoes are inappropriate and potentially dangerous when your are regaining mobility after surgery.

Restrictive clothing may impair the circulation of a swollen limb, and therefore any tight-fitting clothes, such as panty girdles or jeans, should be avoided. They will also be uncomfortable and difficult to get on and off in the first few days after surgery. The elastic around the legs of your underpants should be loose.

3   *Towel and washing things*.

4   *Walking aids/surgical shoes*. You should take in to hospital any walking aids you already use as they may need to be repaired or changed to suit your gait after surgery. People who have

suffered pain and disability prior to hip replacement surgery develop an abnormal gait which will have to be corrected post-operatively. It is therefore important that their walking aids are adapted to suit a more normal way of walking.

If you have been wearing surgical or specially adapted shoes, you should also take these in to hospital with you so that any necessary alterations can be made to them.

5   *Money, jewellery etc.* A *small* amount of money may be useful for newspapers and the telephone. Large sums of money, handbags, wallets and jewellery should not be taken into hospital as these may have to be kept in an unlocked cabinet by your bed. Any valuables or large sums of money you have to take with you should be given to the ward sister for safe keeping when you are admitted. You will be given a receipt listing each item, which you should keep safe so that you can collect your possessions when you are discharged. However, hospital authorities strongly discourage people from bringing anything of great value with them unless absolutely necessary. It is better to make arrangements for any valuables you do not wish to leave at home to be looked after by a relative or friend while you are in hospital.

6   *Books, magazines, puzzles etc.* There will inevitably be periods of waiting between visits from medical staff before your operation, and you may want something to occupy you during this time as well as post-operatively.

7   *Drugs you are already taking.* Once your admission has been arranged, your family doctor will have been asked to fill in a form stating all the drugs you are taking and their doses. You may be asked to take your drugs with you when you are admitted to hospital so that their dosages can be checked and so that you can continue to be given any which are necessary. All your drugs will be kept for you during your stay

as you must only take those which are given to you by medical staff. They should, however, be returned to you before you leave.

8 *Admission letter*. You should take with you the admission letter sent to you from the hospital.

> **Wedding rings** Wedding rings, or any other rings which are very precious to you or which cannot be removed, will be covered with adhesive tape before your operation. This is to prevent the metal causing burns during the process of **electrocautery** (or **diathermy**) which is used to control bleeding during surgery. In electrocautery, an electric current heats the tip of an instrument which is used to shrivel and seal the little blood vessels and stop them bleeding.

HOSPITAL STAFF

The ward of a hospital is a busy place and can seem rather confusing and frightening. It may help to have an idea of the different medical staff you are likely to meet, and the jobs they do.

Nurses

The uniforms worn to distinguish nurses of different ranks will vary from hospital to hospital, but all nurses wear badges which state clearly their name and sometimes their grade. There are, of course, both male and female nurses, although women are still in the majority. The nursing grades are as follows.

1 The most senior nurse on the ward is the *ward sister* or *ward manager*. Each ward will have one ward sister who will be very experienced and able to answer any questions you may have. The ward sister has 24-hour a day responsibility for all the staff and patients on at least one ward, for the day-to-

day running of the ward, standards of care etc., and is ulti-
mately responsible for the ward even when not on duty. She
will be a registered nurse (RN) or a registered general nurse
(RGN), who has usually been qualified for at least five years.
Ward sisters may wear a uniform of a single colour, often
dark blue.

The male equivalent of the ward sister is a *charge nurse*,
whose rank will be clearly displayed on his name badge.
Charge nurses wear a white tunic.

2   When the ward sister is not on duty, there may be a *senior
staff nurse* or a *team leader* of another grade in charge. The
senior staff nurse is deputy to, and works closely with, the
ward sister. Like the ward sister, this nurse will be very
experienced.

3   Each ward may have several *staff nurses* – registered or registered general nurses who have completed their nursing
training. They may be newly qualified or may have several
years' experience, and will take charge of the ward when
both the ward sister and senior staff nurse are unavailable.
There are different grades of staff nurse, distinguished by
different coloured belts, epaulettes, uniforms or, more
rarely nowadays, hats.

The more junior staff nurses are very often in their first or
second post since qualifying. They are less involved in ward
management, and are therefore able to work closely with
the patients.

4   *Enrolled nurses* have undergone two years of training. They are
gradually being replaced and can now undergo a training
programme to become staff nurses with the qualification
RGN. However, there are still many enrolled nurses working
on hospital wards who are very experienced and sometimes
team leaders (see above).

5   As student nurses now spend more time in college and less on the wards of hospitals, *health care assistants* (HCAs) are being brought in to take their place. These are unqualified nurses who have undergone six months' training on day release while working on a ward and who have then been assessed for a National Vocational Qualification (NVQ) by senior nurses. Health care assistants are able to carry out all basic nursing duties except for the dispensing of drugs. They are supervised at all times by a qualified nurse.

6   The ward may also have several *nursing auxiliaries* who are present to deal with any non-medical jobs and to help with the basic care of patients such as making beds, serving tea, and putting away linen etc. Although nursing auxiliaries are not trained nurses, some are very experienced and have acquired greater responsibility.

7   Student nurses – *diploma nursing students* or Project 2000 *students* – are unpaid and allocated to the wards at various stages during their college-based training. They are mainly involved in observing and carrying out limited clinical tasks. In their last term before they qualify, they will be rostered on to nursing shifts and be part of a ward team.

Doctors

Each consultant surgeon in a hospital may head a team of doctors of different ranks, sometimes known as a 'firm'. You may meet some or all of them. These doctors can, of course, be men or women.

1   The *consultant surgeon* holds the ultimate responsibility for all the patients on the operating list, and for the work of all the staff in the 'firm'. Consultants have at least 10 to 15 years' experience as surgeons.

Unless you are being treated privately (see Chapter 12), you may only see the consultant who is responsible for your care at your first out-patient appointment and possibly during a ward round after your operation. Otherwise, you are likely to be seen by a registrar (see below). You should be visited on the ward before your operation by whichever surgeon is to perform it.

2   The *senior registrar* is an experienced surgeon who has completed several years of training and will soon be appointed to a consultant post. (This grade of surgeon is soon to be changed.)

3   Your operation may be performed by a *registrar* rather than by a consultant surgeon or senior registrar. Registrars have trained as surgeons for at least two or three years and are able to carry out some surgery alone, assisting the consultant or being assisted by the consultant on more difficult operations.

4   Some hospitals employ *clinical assistants* as surgeons. These are often very experienced surgeons who, for personal or family reasons, are not able to work full time.

5   You may be examined before your operation by a *senior house officer* (SHO) or by a house surgeon (see below). Senior house officers have been qualified doctors for between one and five years, and are gaining further experience in hospital before becoming surgical registrars or specialising in another branch of medicine.

6   A *house surgeon* (or *house officer*) is likely to be directly concerned with your care both before and after your operation, taking notes of your medical history and arranging for any necessary pre-operative investigations to be done, such as a blood count, chest X-ray and electrocardiogram. House

officers are qualified doctors who have completed at least five years of undergraduate training and are working for a further year in hospital before becoming fully registered. Although house officers do not perform surgery on their own, they may assist the surgeon in the operating theatre.

Anaesthetists are doctors who have been trained in the administration of drugs which cause loss of sensation or consciousness, or both (anaesthetics), and those which block feelings of pain (analgesics). An anaesthetist may visit you before your operation to discuss any relevant details, such as any anaesthetics you have had in the past and any drugs you may be taking (see Chapter 6), and will be present throughout your operation.

ADMISSION TO THE WARD

When you arrive at the hospital, you should report to the main reception desk with your admission letter. The staff there will check your details and tell you which ward to go to. Once on the ward, the ward clerk or a nurse will deal with the clerical side of your admission, filling in the necessary forms with you. You will then be shown to your bed and told of any ward details such as meal times, where to find the toilets, day room etc.

In Britain, the 'Named Nurse Initiative' was introduced under the Government's Patients' Charter. In a National Health Service (NHS) hospital, each patient is allocated a **named nurse** who is responsible for planning that patient's nursing care throughout their stay. The ward sister will, of course, still be informed of all aspects of your care, and will be able to discuss it with you or your relatives.

Your named nurse will admit you to the ward, look after you during your stay, and co-ordinate your discharge when the time comes. Other nurses will be allocated from the team for other working shifts. The idea is for people to be identified as individuals who are known to at least one nurse on each shift and who are involved in their own care. To this end, you may be asked to help your nurse draw up a care plan when you are admitted to the ward. You should tell the nurse of any ailments, preferences or dislikes you have, for example if you prefer to sleep with several pillows or if there are certain foods you do not want.

Your nurse's name may be displayed above your bed or on your bedside locker so that your relatives and other nursing and medical staff know who to talk to about your care. Your care plan may be kept at the bottom of your bed, but wherever it is, it is available for you to read. Nursing staff may tick off a checklist as they carry out the various procedures and will update the care plan with you as the need arises.

Questionnaires Apart from being involved in research of one type or another, hospital staff are always attempting to improve the care they offer. Therefore, on admission to hospital you may be given a questionnaire to fill in before you leave, giving details of the positive and negative aspects of your hospital stay. You will not be asked to sign the form, and can therefore feel free to be honest in your answers without the fear of causing offence. It is very helpful to hospital staff to receive feedback from their patients so that they can be sure they are providing the right service in the right way, and you should try to complete any questionnaire you are given if at all possible.

The nurse will measure your blood pressure, temperature and pulse. A sample of your urine may be taken for analysis and you may be weighed if the anaesthetist needs to know your weight in order to be able to calculate the dose of anaesthetic you require.

Do tell a nurse if you have any problems or if you are anxious about *any* aspect of your hospital stay.

Clinical trials To be able to improve the treatment given to people, new therapies need to be tested, and currently used treatment regimes need to be tried in different ways. Therefore you may be asked to take part in a clinical trial to compare a new treatment with an existing one.

The details of any trial will be explained to you, and you should make sure you fully understand what is entailed before you make a decision. Once you understand the implications of the trial, and if you agree to be included, you will be asked to sign a consent form. You are under no obligation to take part in a clinical trial and, if you refuse, the quality of the treatment you receive will not be affected in any way.

THROMBOSIS PREVENTION

Normally, the activity of the muscles in the legs helps to keep the blood moving through them. During long periods of bed rest or anaesthesia, these muscles are inactive and the circulation of blood in the legs slows down. A blood clot – known as a **thrombus** – is thus more likely to form and can block the passage of blood through the vein, causing a **thrombosis**. If a piece of the blood clot breaks off, it forms an **embolus** which may travel through the circulation and lodge in a vital organ such as the lung, causing a **pulmonary embolism**, with serious consequences (see p.89).

Thrombosis is relatively common after any type of pelvic surgery, including hip replacement, and precautions will be taken to try to reduce the risk.

Anti-embolism stockings

Once you are settled on the ward, a nurse will measure your legs for anti-embolism stockings (often called TEDS – **t**hrombo-

embolic **d**eterrent **s**tockings). These stockings are used routinely in some hospitals, and are invariably worn by anyone having a hip replacement operation and whose mobility will be limited to some degree for several weeks. They help prevent blood clots forming in the deep veins of the legs by improving the return of blood to the heart. Although the stockings may feel a bit uncomfortable, particularly when the weather is hot, there is no doubt as to their value.

Once you have had a bath or shower and are getting ready to leave the ward for your operation, an anti-embolism stocking will probably be put on the leg which is not being operated on. Another stocking will be put on the operated leg the morning after your operation. You will have to wear both stockings for about six weeks. When necessary, they should be washed during the day while you are mobile, and dried to wear again at night when the risk of thrombosis is greater. They should not, however, be dried over direct heat, such as on a radiator, as it will reduce their elasticity and therefore their effectiveness.

Foot pumps

You may be given special boots to wear while you are in bed after your operation. These boots are designed to reduce the risk of deep vein thrombosis. They are made of a soft, foam-like material and attached to a foot pump at the end of the bed. A pocket under each foot systematically inflates and deflates, assisting the circulation of blood in the legs. If you are given foot pumps, they will probably be kept on whenever you are in bed throughout your stay in hospital. A member of the medical staff will help you to take them off and put them on again when your want to get out of and into bed. Although the value of these foot pumps is still being assessed, they are already used routinely in some hospitals.

Heparin injections

You may also be given injections of low-dose heparin through-out your stay in hospital to reduce the risk of blood clots form-ing. Heparin is an anticoagulant which occurs naturally in the body, thinning the blood and helping to prevent it from clotting. (Higher doses of heparin, or of a similar substance called war-farin, can be given to treat a blood clot once it has developed.) Heparin injections are not given routinely in all hospitals, but they are invariably necessary for anyone at particular risk of thrombosis.

VISIT BY A DOCTOR

As has already been mentioned, a house surgeon or senior house officer will visit you on the ward before your operation to take details of your medical history – including any allergies you may have and any drugs you are taking – and to examine you. Your family doctor may have already filled in a form giving the names and dosages of any drugs you have been prescribed, and you should have been told what to do about these. Do not for-get to tell the hospital doctor of any other drugs you have been taking which your family doctor may not be aware of, such as vit-amin supplements, cough medicines, aspirins etc., which are available from a pharmacy without the need for prescription.

A medical examination will be carried out to detect any ill-ness or infection you may have which could complicate the use of a general anaesthetic. You may also have a chest X-ray, an electrocardiogram, a urine test and a blood test, even if you have already attended a pre-operative assessment clinic. If you have rheumatoid arthritis, an X-ray may be taken of your neck to make sure you have sufficient movement in it to enable the anaesthetist to insert a tube through your mouth during anaesthesia.

The surgeon who is to perform your operation may also visit you on the ward to check that all is well. If you have not already done so, you will be asked to sign a consent form.

VISIT BY THE ANAESTHETIST

An anaesthetist will probably come to see you before your operation to discuss anything that may be relevant to the choice of anaesthetic given to you. Do make sure that you mention any aspect of your anaesthesia which causes you concern so that the anaesthetist can explain things to you and put your mind at rest. For example, many people are anxious about anaesthetics being administered through a face mask. Although face masks are now not normally used until patients are sedated, it is worth mentioning this fear so that your anaesthetist is aware of it and can reassure you.

Pre-medication

Anaesthetics have improved considerably during the last few years, and a 'pre-med.' is now not always given routinely. However, if you enter hospital the day before your operation and think that you will be too anxious to sleep that night, do ask the house surgeon or senior house officer for something to help you.

Sometimes spinal and epidural anaesthetics (see Chapter 6) are injected in the operating theatre while the patient is sitting on the edge of the operating table, supported by a nurse. In these cases, sedation with a pre-med. is not appropriate as patients need to be alert and able to comply with simple instructions while the injection is administered. Some people are upset if they expect to have a pre-med. and are told they cannot have one, and it is best to be prepared in advance for this possibility.

If you are having a pre-med., it will be given to you an hour or two before your operation to sedate you. If it is routine practice in your hospital for everyone to have a pre-med., do tell the anaesthetist if you prefer to do without one.

False teeth

You should tell the anaesthetist if you have any false teeth or dental bridges as these will have to be removed before you go into the operating theatre. A broken or loose tooth can be inhaled into the lungs during surgery. You should also point out any teeth which are crowned. In some hospitals you will be able to wear your false teeth until you reach the operating theatre rather than having to take them out on the ward.

VISITS BY OTHER MEDICAL STAFF

It is sometimes routine practice for operating theatre staff to visit people on the ward before their operations to explain theatre procedures and equipment to them. You may also be introduced to a nurse from the recovery room, possibly when you are taken to the operating theatre. These visits are made in an attempt to reduce some of the anxiety associated with surgery by introducing people to the nurses who will care for them during and immediately after their operation.

Medical social workers

If any problems arise at home during your stay in hospital, or if you are concerned about being able to manage on your own once you are discharged, you can ask to talk to a medical social worker. Medical social workers work in close partnership with other medical staff in the hospital and will be able to give you advice and practical support. If necessary, you may be kept in hospital a little longer than normal until nursing staff are happy that you will be able to manage or that arrangements have been made to help you once you are at home.

It is important that enough time is allowed to make arrangements for any necessary assistance once you leave hospital, and you should therefore make known any potential problems as soon as possible, ideally at your pre-operative assessment appointment.

Physiotherapists

A physiotherapist is someone who is trained to assist patients to rehabilitate following illness, injury or deformity. You may have been referred to a physiotherapist some time before your operation if you needed special treatment such as hydrotherapy for a particular problem.

A physiotherapist may visit you on the ward before your operation to assess your mobility and any problems you have, such as deformity or loss of use of other joints due, for example, to rheumatoid arthritis, which could affect the post-operative exercises you are able to do, or the way you do them. This visit is useful in that it allows the physiotherapist to plan an exercise routine tailored to your individual needs.

During the physiotherapist's visit, you may also be shown how to do some simple exercises immediately after your operation, such as ankle movements to assist your circulation while you are immobile in bed (see p.64). The physiotherapist may ask you to try to lift your bottom off the bed by pushing yourself up using your good leg. The ability to do this will enable you to change your position in bed after your operation, to make yourself more comfortable and to help to avoid pressure sores. If you cannot change your position in this way, a special **monkey pole** may be attached above your bed for you to hold onto.

The physiotherapist will discuss with you the importance of

deep breathing to help reduce the risk of chest problems post-operatively, and may show you some breathing exercises. He or she will probably already be aware of any specific problems you have which may affect your post-operative rehabilitation, and may talk to you about these. Your rehabilitation programme will also be explained to you, as will the precautions you will have to take post-operatively to avoid dislocating your new hip (see p.70).

PREPARING FOR SURGERY

There are several routine procedures which will take place in the hours before your operation.

'Nil by mouth'

This is a term which means that neither food nor drink must be swallowed. In order to prevent vomiting and the risk of choking on your vomit while you are anaesthetised, you may be told not to eat or drink anything for four to six hours before your oper-ation, although you will be able to have a few sips of water with any tablets you need to take. Even people having an epidural or spinal anaesthetic will be given some sort of sedation during their operation, and it is always possible that surgery started with a spinal or epidural anaesthetic may have to be completed using general anaesthesia. Therefore, whatever type of anaes-thetic you are due to have, you will be 'nil by mouth' in the pre-ceding hours, although some anaesthetists now allow their patients to drink clear fluids up to three hours pre-operatively.

Bathing

You may be told to have a bath or shower a couple of hours or more before your operation, either during the morning of the same day or the night before. You can use ordinary soap and water but should not use deodorant, talcum powder, nail varnish, perfume etc.

Shaving

The operation site is unlikely to be shaved before hip surgery. Although shaving used to be routine practice, it is now thought that it has the potential to increase the risk of infection post-operatively.

Smoking

If you are a heavy smoker and have not been able to cut down or stop altogether, you will be advised not to smoke in the hours before your operation. It is, of course, much better to stop smoking some months before surgery, and some surgeons will not perform non-emergency operations on heavy smokers. The carbon monoxide contained in cigarette smoke poisons the blood by replacing some of the oxygen which is carried in it and which is vital to processes such as wound healing. Smoking also increases the risk of chest infection post-operatively.

Waiting

As already mentioned, you are likely to be admitted to hospital at least the day before your operation so that any necessary tests and examinations can be done and their results received and so that the medical staff mentioned above can visit you on the ward.

Occasionally surgery has to be cancelled at the last moment because an emergency has arisen and an earlier operation has taken longer than expected or has met with complications. If this does occur, you may be sent home and called again at the earliest opportunity. Although this would obviously be distressing, do try not to get upset. Other operations taking place on the same day may be more urgent than yours and unable to be postponed. In the UK, under the terms of the Patients' Charter, a cancelled operation must be done within one month, and the medical staff will certainly make every effort to do yours as soon as possible.

You will probably be given only an approximate time for your operation.

Leaving the ward for your operation

Before being taken from the ward to the anaesthetic room or operating theatre, the hip to be operated on will be marked with a felt-tip pen. You may be asked several times by different medical staff – possibly including the surgeon – which hip is to be operated on. Do not be worried by this question; it does not mean that they do not know! Repeated checks of this sort help to avoid mistakes being made, which are possible when so many operations are done each day in a large and busy hospital.

You will be given a hospital operating gown to wear; a plastic-covered bracelet bearing your name and an identifying hospital number will be attached to one or each of your wrists; and an anti-embolism stocking will be put on your 'good' leg. You will then leave the ward on a hospital trolley.

If you have a hearing aid, it will probably be removed once you are asleep and replaced in the recovery room.

The anaesthetic room

In the anaesthetic room, a small tube called a **cannula** will be inserted into a vein in the back of your hand. The cannula will be kept in place throughout the operation to provide a channel for the administration of drugs. The anaesthetic will probably be administered in the anaesthetic room, although it may be given in the operating theatre itself. A general anaesthetic will take effect within seconds, a spinal or epidural anaesthetic within a matter of minutes. Once the anaesthetist is satisfied that you are properly anaesthetised, you are ready for your operation.

CHAPTER 6

Anaesthesia for surgery

This chapter describes the different anaesthetics used for hip replacement operations. The anaesthetic chosen for you may depend on the type of operation you are having and on the normal practice of your anaesthetist. It may be possible for your own preferences to be taken into account, if you have any, so do discuss them with the anaesthetist during the ward visit.

REGIONAL ANAESTHESIA

Regional anaesthesia is sometimes used, usually in combination with a sedative to put you to sleep. It is a form of local anaesthesia for which the anaesthetic drug is contained within a specific area of the body. You may be given one of two types, either a spinal or an epidural. Sometimes a tracheal tube is inserted to keep the airways open, in which case you may also be given a very light general anaesthetic to enable the tube to be passed down your throat.

Spinal anaesthesia

For a spinal anaesthetic, the drug is injected between the vertebrae of the spine into the space around the nerves in the back. It causes numbness in the legs and groin which lasts for between one and a half and three hours, or longer in older people. The anaesthetic takes effect within about five minutes, causing the legs and lower body to become numb and heavy. Spread of the drug can be controlled within the desired area by the addition of glucose to make it heavier and by appropriate positioning of your body during the operation.

Spinal anaesthetics induce profound muscle relaxation and can be used in low doses, thus avoiding any complications of toxicity. However, they can cause headaches and have a limited duration of action.

Epidural anaesthesia

Epidural anaesthesia is similar to spinal anaesthesia and is sometimes used for hip operations. The anaesthetic drug is injected into the back but, unlike for a spinal anaesthetic, the needle does not penetrate the membrane around the spinal cord (the **dura**). The effects of an epidural last longer than those of a spinal anaesthetic and epidurals can therefore provide pain relief for a period after surgery.

A small tube called a **catheter** is inserted into the back and left in place throughout the operation so that additional doses of the drug can be introduced as required. The catheter is sometimes retained for a day or two after surgery so that pain-killing drugs can be administered through it.

Epidural anaesthetics take 15 minutes or more to have an effect.

GENERAL ANAESTHESIA

Most hip replacement operations are done using general anaesthesia. A general anaesthetic will put you to sleep so that you have no feeling in any part of your body. It may be an **intravenous anaesthetic**, injected into a vein in your hand or arm through a plastic tube, or an **inhalational anaesthetic** in the form of a gas which you breathe in. In fact, both types are normally used, although you will probably only be aware of the injection which sends you off to sleep.

If you are having a general anaesthetic, you may be visited on the ward by an anaesthetist before your operation. The main reason for this visit is to decide what type of anaesthesia would be safest for you. It also gives you the opportunity to discuss any problems or worries you may have. The anaesthetist will ask you several questions about any anaesthetics you have had before, any drugs you are taking, and about your general health. It is important that you answer these questions as fully as possible. You should also mention to the anaesthetist if you have any false or crowned teeth.

If you have had problems in the past such as an allergy to a particular anaesthetic, it will be helpful if you know the name of the drug concerned and/or the hospital where the operation was carried out. The appropriate records can then be checked to make sure another type of anaesthetic is used. You should also tell the anaesthetist if you know of any other member of your family who has reacted against a particular drug, as you may have the same problem.

Risks of general anaesthesia

Some people are afraid of being put to sleep by a general anaesthetic, but the risk is small. Advances in anaesthesia over the past few years have been tremendous. Although complications still occasionally occur and, very rarely, people do suffer brain damage or even die during surgery – risks which do need to be borne in mind – you are far more likely to be killed in a road accident than to suffer any serious ill-effect from the use of an anaesthetic.

Careful consideration will be given by the surgeon and anaesthetist to your general state of health and all other relevant factors before deciding to go ahead with your operation and anaesthesia. People with certain medical conditions, such as serious heart or lung disease, may not be given general anaesthetics as they are potentially at greater risk. However, if you are worried about any risks involved, do discuss your concerns with the anaesthetist.

During your operation

Several different types of drugs will be given to you during your operation:

* *induction agents* to bring on sleep;

* *maintenance agents* to keep you asleep;

* *analgesics* to stop you feeling pain after the operation;

* *anti-emetics* to help stop you feeling sick after the operation;

* *muscle relaxants*.

Analgesics and anti-emetics are also given post-operatively as required.

When the operation is over, the anaesthetist will stop giving you the drugs that were keeping you asleep, and you will be taken to a recovery room (see p.54).

Side-effects of general anaesthesia

There are some side-effects related to the use of general anaesthetics, but these are usually minor and do not last very long. The most common are nausea and vomiting. You may also have a sore throat after your operation, possibly due to the 'dry' anaesthetic gases used to keep you asleep during surgery, or to the tube which may have been placed in your throat to maintain an airway and help you to breathe. Whatever the reason, any soreness usually disappears after two or three days and can be eased by simple painkillers. The muscle relaxants used during anaesthesia can cause muscle aches and pains, which should improve within about 48 hours.

OTHER MEDICATION

The anaesthetist will explain about other tablets and drugs which may be required before your operation. You may be given the option of having a 'pre-med.', usually in the form of tablets given one to two hours before surgery. If you are anxious about your operation, you may wish to ask for a 'pre-med.' if their use is not routine in your hospital.

The anaesthetist will also explain about any antibiotics or anticoagulants (blood-thinning drugs) you may require. Drugs which you normally take, such as diuretics ('water tablets') or drugs to reduce high blood pressure, may also be continued but you must only take those which are given to you by medical staff.

BEFORE YOUR OPERATION

You will probably be told not to have anything to eat or drink for about six hours before your operation ('nil by mouth'). If you are having a 'pre-med.', it may be given to you while you are still on the ward, and you will soon begin to feel sleepy. There is no need to be alarmed: the 'pre-med.' is not an anaesthetic itself, it is only to relax you and stop you feeling anxious.

When you are taken from the ward, you may go first to the anaesthetic room or straight to the operating theatre to be given your anaesthetic. The anaesthetist, or an assistant, will fit some monitoring devices to watch over you while you are asleep. These may include a little probe which goes on your finger to measure the amount of oxygen in your blood, an electrocardiogram (ECG) to observe your heart beat, and a cuff around your arm to measure your blood pressure. Once the anaesthetist is happy with the readings from these monitors, the anaesthesia will start.

If you are having a general anaesthetic, a cannula will be put into a vein in the back of your hand or arm, and the anaesthetic drugs will be introduced into your body through it. Once the anaesthetic has been injected, you will fall asleep within seconds. The drug which makes you go to sleep may sting a little as it enters the vein from the cannula, but this feeling does not last long. For a spinal or epidural anaesthetic, you will be asked to sit on the edge of the bed or trolley or to lie on your side while the drug is injected into your back.

The anaesthetist will remain with you throughout the operation to make sure you are asleep and that the function of your heart and lungs is satisfactory.

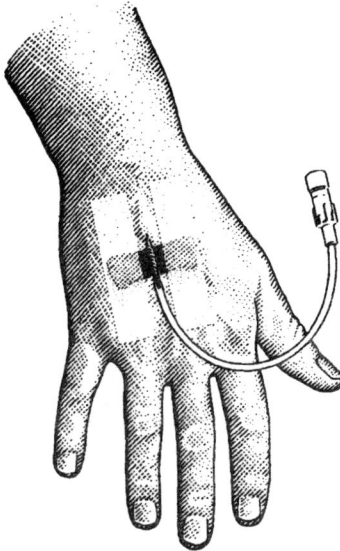

A cannula. The cannula is inserted into a vein in the back of the hand to allow the flow of anaesthetic drugs to be controlled during surgery.

THE RECOVERY ROOM

The nurses in the recovery room are specially trained to care for patients coming round from anaesthetics after an operation. You will stay in this room, still watched over by monitoring equipment, until you are fully awake and ready to be returned to your own ward.

If you are in any pain when you wake up, the staff in the recovery room will be able to give you something to relieve it. This can be an injection through the cannula which is already in place or directly into your arm or leg. If you have had a spinal or epidural anaesthetic, the catheter will probably still be in your back so that pain-killing drugs can be introduced through it as required.

PAIN RELIEF

When you return to your ward, the house surgeon and nurses will be able to give you analgesics for any pain. However, if these are not enough, do ask the anaesthetist or ward staff for something more effective.

The amount of discomfort suffered after any operation varies from person to person, and of course depends on the extent of the surgery involved.

Patient-controlled analgesia

In some hospitals, patient-controlled analgesia (PCA) may be offered after a hip operation, but PCA machines are expensive and may not be available for all patients. The PCA technique has been designed to allow patients themselves to control the amount of analgesic they receive, and it is generally a more effective way of providing pain relief than the conventional forms.

The machine is basically a pump which delivers a pain-killing drug into your body each time you press a button. It is programmed to allow you only a safe limit of the drug, which is usually delivered via a cannula in a vein in your hand or arm. When you press the button, your pain should start to reduce within five to ten minutes. If it does not do so, press the button again. As the machine has a built-in safety control to prevent you receiving too much of the drug, you can press the button as often as you like. However, it is important that you do not let anyone else use your machine as doing so would remove the safety feature. If, despite pressing the button several times, your pain is not being relieved, tell a nurse or doctor as it may be possible for the machine to be reset to deliver a stronger dose of the drug.

A nurse or doctor will inspect the counter on your machine every hour or so to see how many times you have pressed the button and how much analgesic drug you have received. Once it is clear that you are reducing the amount of drug you need, and therefore your pain is improving, the machine setting will be changed to deliver a lower dose at each press of the button. When patient-controlled analgesia is needed, it can normally be replaced with analgesic tablets after 24 to 48 hours.

CHAPTER 7

The operations

This chapter gives brief details of the two main types of hip surgery: total hip replacement and hemi-arthroplasty. The latter is usually done following fracture of the hip just below the head of the femur, a relatively common injury in the elderly.

TOTAL HIP REPLACEMENT

Once the anaesthetic has taken effect, you will be positioned on the operating table on your back or on your side, depending on the surgeon's preference. If you are placed on your side, you will be supported by bolsters in front and behind you.

Your leg will then be cleaned with antiseptic and your whole body, except for the operation site, will be covered with sterile drapes. An adherent film of plastic sheeting will be placed over the operation site itself to isolate the wound from the surrounding skin. These precautions are necessary to reduce the risk of introducing infection into the wound.

The surgeon will make an incision in the skin overlying the hip, probably at the side through the gluteal muscles (see p.5) or posteriorly from behind these muscles. The capsule which surrounds the hip joint will be opened and the hip dislocated. The head of the femur (the ball part of the joint) can then be excised and the acetabulum (the cup part) exposed.

Any residual cartilage and hard bone are ground away with an instrument called a **reamer**. If a cemented acetabular cup is

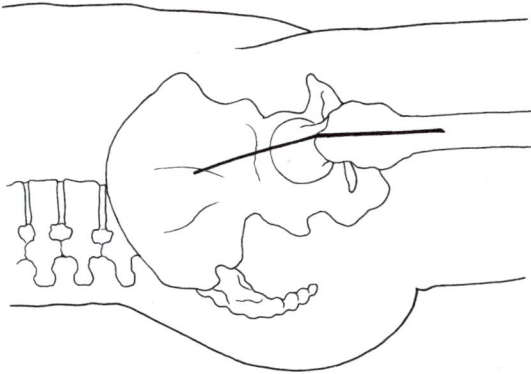

A lateral skin incision, often used for total hip replacement.

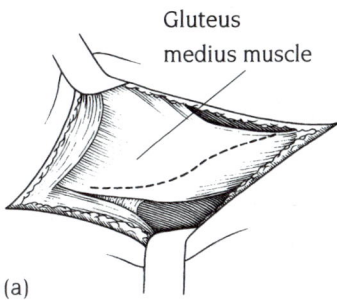

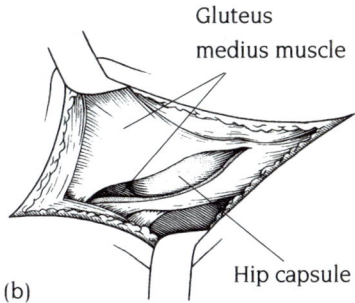

Gluteus medius muscle

Gluteus medius muscle

Hip capsule

(a)

(b)

Muscle incision following a lateral skin incision. Once the skin has been cut: (a) the gluteus medius muscle is incised along the line indicated, and (b) the hip capsule is exposed.

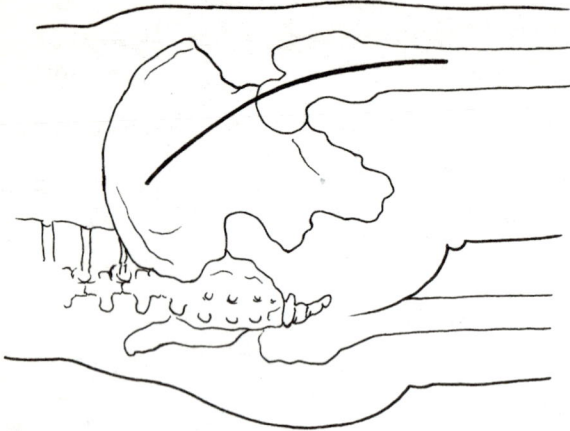

A postero-lateral skin incision. Another type of skin incision some-times used for total hip replacement.

being inserted, holes will be made in the adjacent bone and the bone itself will be cleaned and dried before the plastic cup is cemented into position. A cementless acetabular cup will be slightly bigger than the hole which has been carefully prepared to take it, and its surface will be roughened.

The marrow cavity in the neck of the thigh bone will be pre-pared for the insertion of the femoral component, and a restric-tor inserted into it to prevent cement seeping down towards the knee. The marrow cavity is cleaned and dried before the cement is introduced into it under pressure. A specially selected femoral component can then be inserted into the cement, which sets within seven to ten minutes of mixing. Although many femoral prostheses are in one piece, with the head attached to the stem, modern ones often have two separate parts so that a head of the

(a)

Gluteus maximus
muscle

Fascia lata

(b)

Sciatic nerve

Quadratus femoris

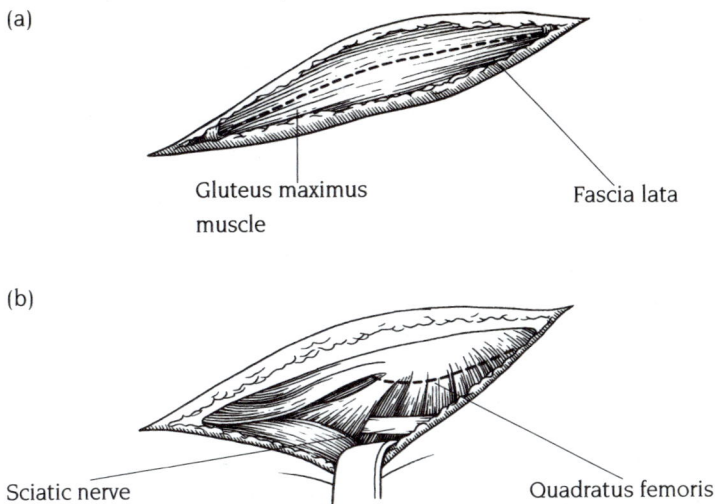

Muscle incision following a postero-lateral skin incision. (a) The gluteus maximus muscle is cut along the line indicated. (b) The quadratus femoris muscle can then be incised (along the dashed line) to reveal the hip capsule.

correct length can be attached to the stem once it has been cemented into the bone.

The hip will then be restored to its normal position (**reduced**) and taken through a full range of movement to test the stability of the joint. If the joint is stable, the surgeon will stitch the muscles back in place and use an absorbable suture material to close the outer layers of tissue which lie between the hip joint and the skin. Two suction drains are normally inserted into the deeper layers of tissue to drain away any blood which may collect. The skin will then be closed with non-absorbable sutures, or with clips, and a pressure dressing will be applied.

After this operation, the legs are often strapped to an abduction pillow to keep them apart. Although there is always some risk that the new hip joint could become dislocated, particularly before it has healed and stabilised, the danger is greatest in the first few hours after surgery, especially during the period of recovery from anaesthesia when people are often rather confused. An abduction pillow may therefore be kept in place for 24 hours post-operatively.

When you leave the operating theatre, you will be taken to the recovery room to come round from the anaesthetic.

HEMI-ARTHROPLASTY

Once the anaesthetic has taken effect, you will be positioned on the operating table, on your side and supported by bolsters. Your leg will be cleaned and covered with sterile drapes, leaving only the operation site exposed.

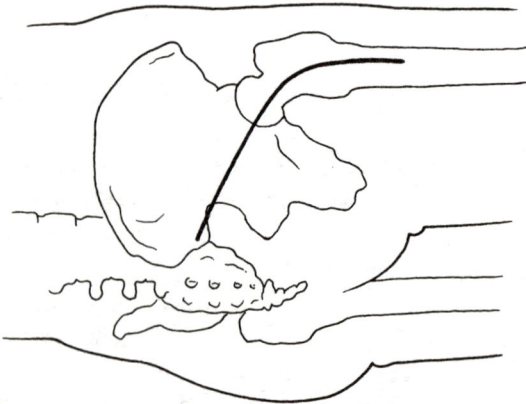

A posterior skin incision, used for hemi-arthroplasty and sometimes for total hip replacement.

The surgeon will make an incision over the outer surface of your hip, curving backwards onto the buttock, and the muscles at the back of the hip will be detached to expose the hip joint. As this operation is done following fracture through the neck of the thigh bone, the head of the bone (the ball) will still be in place in the acetabulum (the cup or socket of the joint), and a corkscrew is often used to remove it. The size of the femoral head which has been removed will be measured so that a prosthesis of similar size can be selected. The upper part of the remainder of the thigh bone will then be prepared by reaming (see above), the prosthesis inserted into it, and the hip restored to its normal position. The stability of the hip will then be tested by taking it through a full range of movement.

The surgeon will stitch the muscles at the back of the hip into place, insert suction drains, and suture the overlying tissues and skin.

Once the operation is complete, you will be taken to the recovery room and monitored until you wake up and are fit to be returned to your ward.

CHAPTER 8

After your operation: in hospital

When you come round from the anaesthetic, you will be taken from the recovery room back to your hospital ward. You may have been put back onto your own bed in the operating theatre while still anaesthetised and will be lying flat on your back with your legs held apart by a wedge or pillow. Although this position can be a bit uncomfortable, it is necessary to help avoid dislocation of your new hip joint.

In the past, people stayed in hospital (mostly in bed) for about four weeks after hip surgery. Post-operative care and surgical techniques have changed dramatically in recent years, and you may be in hospital for between five days and two weeks, being encouraged to become mobile again as soon as possible. Procedures and normal practice vary from hospital to hospital. This chapter gives a general idea of what to expect during your hospital stay, but you will be given specific instructions and advice by medical staff.

EXERCISES TO DO IN BED

Whether or not you were advised to do some simple exercises before your operation, you should start them as soon as possible when you are back on the ward – *unless you are told otherwise for some reason*. If at any time you find it painful to do the exercises you have been told to do, you should stop doing them immediately and ask your physiotherapist's or doctor's advice.

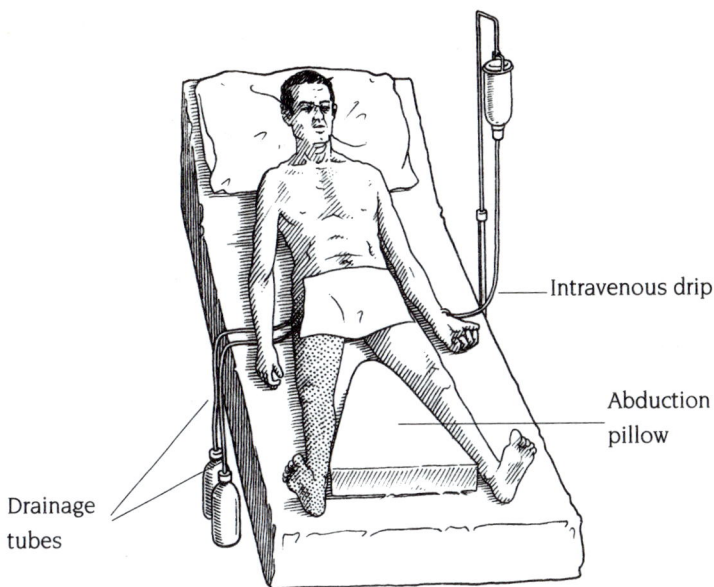

Intravenous drip

Abduction
pillow

Drainage
tubes

Coming round after your operation. When you wake up after surgery you will be lying on your back with your legs held apart by an abduction pillow. There will be one or more drainage tubes inserted near your wound to drain away the excess blood and fluid, and an intravenous drip in your arm to replace the fluid (or blood) lost during your operation. (The operated leg is shaded.)

Deep breathing

You may be given oxygen via a face mask immediately after your operation to assist wound healing if your breathing is shallow. Deep breathing and coughing will help to keep your lungs supplied with oxygen and clear of sputum. If you are at particular risk of chest infection or have a respiratory complaint, a physiotherapist will advise you about some exercises to do.

Leg exercises

Some simple leg exercises will help to reduce the risk of deep vein thrombosis and can easily be done while you are still immobile in bed. Some of them will also help mobilise your hip joint and strengthen your leg muscles. A physiotherapist will probably visit you during the day after your operation and will give you precise instructions about which exercises to do.

1   Flex and extend your feet towards and away from your body and rotate them at the ankles in circular movements. These exercises should preferably be done for at least two minutes every hour.

2   Lying on your back (as you will be after your operation), press your knees onto the bed with your legs straight.

3   Bend your knee and lift it carefully towards your chest. As it is important that the thigh of your operated leg and your body do not come closer than to form an L shape, you should not attempt to bring your knee *close* to your chest when doing this exercise.

PAIN RELIEF

Before you are returned to the ward, you will be given an analgesic (pain-killing) injection containing morphine. If you have had an epidural anaesthetic, the catheter in your back may be kept in place for a couple of days so that morphine can be infused through it. Otherwise, you will be given intramuscular analgesic injections, possibly hourly if your blood pressure and other vital signs remain stable, or you will be provided with a machine to deliver your own patient-controlled analgesia (see p.54) as required. As morphine can induce sickness, you will also have anti-emetic injections to help counteract this effect.

After the first couple of post-operative days, regular analgesic tablets will probably provide sufficient pain relief. You are likely to need to continue taking painkillers for several weeks to enable you to do the necessary exercises. While in hospital, do tell a doctor or nurse if your pain is not being controlled as it may be possible to give you something stronger.

THROMBOSIS PREVENTION

Blood clots are most common about two days after hip surgery, although they can develop anytime up to three weeks or later.

You will continue to wear anti-embolism stockings throughout your stay in hospital and possibly for up to six weeks until the risk of deep vein thrombosis has receded. You may also be given daily injections of a low-dose anticoagulant such as heparin until you leave hospital, although their use is not generally routine except for people who are at particular risk of thrombosis. Occasionally, these injections are continued at home, administered each day by a district nurse.

EATING AND DRINKING

You are unlikely to feel like eating anything until the day after your operation. It is best to have only sips of water for the first few post-operative hours as drinking too much immediately after surgery can make any feeling of sickness worse. Once you do feel like eating again, you will be able to have a light diet for the next day or two, eating normally as soon as you want to.

Drips

When you regain consciousness after surgery, there may be an intravenous drip in your arm for the 24-hour administration of antibiotics and to provide a specially balanced solution to replace the fluids which were lost from your body during the operation.

The drip can usually be taken down after 24 hours, as soon as you are able to eat and drink normally, although it may be kept in place longer if you are likely to need a blood transfusion.

WOUND DRESSINGS AND DRAINS

The wound in your thigh is likely to be 15 to 20 cm (6 to 8 inches) long, or more – much larger than some people expect. There may be one or more small tubes extending out of the side of the wound dressing, possibly held in place with a stitch and draining into a bag or bottle. These drainage tubes enable excess fluid and blood to drain away from the wound, and are removed when wound leakage reduces, usually within about 48 hours. Their removal can be uncomfortable.

There will be a protective dressing over the wound in your thigh which will be checked regularly and changed as required. If your wound is still covered when you leave hospital, arrangements will be made for a district or community nurse to visit you at home to change the dressing.

STITCHES

Your wound may have been closed with staples, clips or stitches. Staples and clips can usually be removed after about seven days and replaced with adhesive strips to support the wound edges until healing is complete. Stitches will probably need to remain in place for 10 to 12 days and, if you have already left hospital by this time, can be removed by a district nurse at your home.

TESTS AND EXAMINATIONS

For the first couple of days after your operation, you will probably have a cuff around your arm, attached to a machine which takes regular readings of your blood pressure. The cuff inflates automatically (which may be a little uncomfortable) at preset intervals – probably every quarter of an hour to begin with and then every half an hour. Each blood pressure reading remains displayed until the next measurement is taken. There may also be a thermometer under your arm to measure your body temperature in the same way. Nursing staff can thus check your blood pressure and temperature as required to monitor your condition.

Although the body temperature is often raised for a few days after surgery, a consistently raised temperature may indicate an infection, the cause of which will need to be investigated. Some people are **hypothermic** (i.e. have a low body temperature) immediately after surgery, and if necessary can be wrapped in a foil blanket for an hour or two to bring their temperature back to normal. A high temperature post-operatively can usually be reduced by placing a fan beside your bed.

The following tests will probably be done during the first post-operative day.

Blood tests

A sample of your blood will be taken the morning after your operation to measure its haemoglobin level. If the haemoglobin is low, you may be started on a course of iron tablets. Blood transfusions are sometimes required if the level of haemoglobin is significantly reduced.

X-rays

An X-ray will be taken of your hip, either before you leave the operating theatre or within 48 hours post-operatively. You may be kept in bed until this has been done, although if there are no signs of any problems, you may be able to get out of bed – but only with assistance – before an X-ray has been taken. The X-ray will be kept for comparison with any taken later so that any changes can be detected.

BLADDER FUNCTION

Until you are able to get out of bed and walk to the toilet, you will be given a bedpan as required.

Urinary problems can sometimes occur in the immediate post-operative period. For example, epidurals often cause urinary retention: the bladder is unable to empty spontaneously and becomes full of urine which cannot be expelled. If this occurs, you are likely to be given antibiotics to reduce the risk of infection, and to have a catheter inserted through your urethra and into your bladder to drain the urine from it. The urinary catheter will probably remain in place until you are mobile and can urinate voluntarily again.

Epidural analgesia, which causes loss of sensation in the lower body, can result in temporary incontinence. If this occurs, a urinary catheter may be inserted to drain your bladder, probably for 48 to 72 hours.

THE PHYSIOTHERAPIST

You will probably be visited on the ward by one or more physiotherapists on the day after your operation, but it is unlikely to be until the next day that you will be helped to get out of bed and to take your first steps using a walking frame .

The team of physiotherapists will be involved in helping you to recover mobility, both by exercising and by practising various activities of daily living. They will also explain which movements and positions you should avoid, and how to use your hip correctly. In unfamiliar surroundings and following anaesthesia, many people find it difficult to concentrate fully in the first few days after an operation, and therefore the information given to

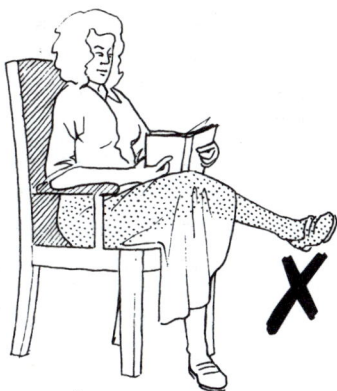

(a)

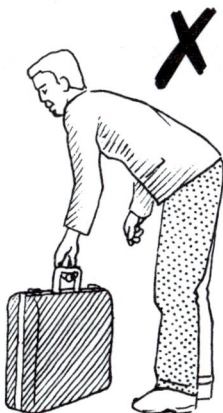

(c)

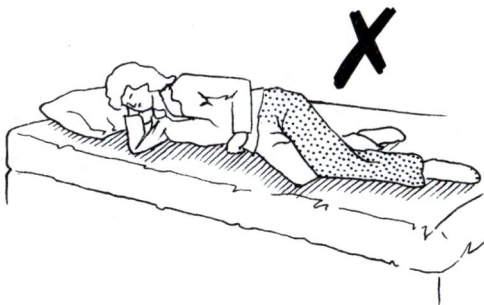

(b)

Precautions to avoid dislocating your new hip. NEVER: (a) cross your legs, (b) lie on your side (for at least a couple of months after your operation), or (c) bend from the waist.

you by your physiotherapist may be repeated several times while you are in hospital.

The physiotherapist will make an assessment of your pattern of gait both before and after your operation and will draw up a programme of exercises – to do in hospital and at home – tailored to your individual needs, age and level of activity.

If you have had hip problems for many months (or even years) before your operation, you will have developed an abnormal gait and length of stride which will need to be corrected post-operatively. The height of any walking aids you use may also have to be adjusted. The physiotherapist will give you clear instructions about any exercises you need to do, and will make sure that you are doing them correctly while in hospital. It is important that you get them right and continue them at home, so if there is anything you do not understand, do ask the physiotherapist to explain it to you again.

Avoiding dislocation The following precautions are important to avoid dislocating your new hip, particularly during the weeks following surgery while the soft tissues are healing and stabilising the joint. They will probably be repeated several times while you are in hospital, by doctors, nurses, physiotherapists and occupational therapists. It may be difficult to remember these restrictions at first, but for most people they gradually become second nature.

Never cross your legs. This rule applies both when sitting and when lying down.

Never bend beyond 90 degrees. The angle between your thigh and the trunk of your body should never be less than 90 degrees, i.e. an L shape. This means avoiding bending down while standing or sitting and avoiding raising your operated leg towards your chest.

Never twist the operated hip. You should never turn your operated leg either outwards or inwards: your toes and knee should always point forward. Nor should you twist your body, for example by reaching across yourself to get something from the locker next to your hospital bed, or by turning from the waist to look behind you.

Hip classes

The physiotherapists at some hospitals hold hip classes once or more a week during which patients are reminded of the 'dos and don'ts' to aid recovery. You may be asked to attend one of these classes once you are reasonably mobile, possibly by the fifth or sixth post-operative day.

GETTING OUT OF BED

Your legs are likely to seem weak to begin with and you may feel dizzy or faint when you first get up. It is therefore important not to attempt to get out of bed without the assistance of a physiotherapist or nurse for the first day or so at least. If you have an epidural for pain relief or patient-controlled analgesia, getting you up will be delayed until it has been removed.

When the physiotherapist(s) helps you to get out of bed, do say immediately if you feel dizzy as it is much easier and safer to put you back onto the bed before you actually faint.

The physiotherapist(s) will help you to sit up, with your weight on your bottom. Keeping your operated leg straight and pivoting on your bottom rather than turning your body or twisting your hip, you will then be able to lift both legs over the side of the bed. Once you are sitting on the edge of the bed, put the foot of your **un**operated leg on the floor, with the knee bent – still keeping your operated leg straight.

Then, using your hands to push yourself up from sitting to standing, slide your operated leg back – still straight – until it is in position on the floor and you feel secure and have gained your balance. This is the point at which you may feel dizzy. If you do, tell the physiotherapist immediately so that you can sit down again. Once you are standing, you can hold the walking frame which will have been put in position in front of you.

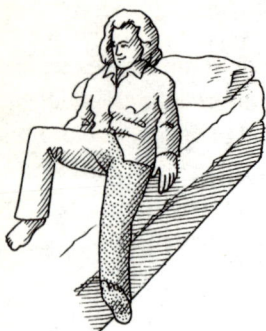

(a)

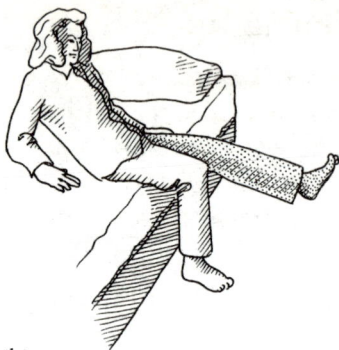

(b)

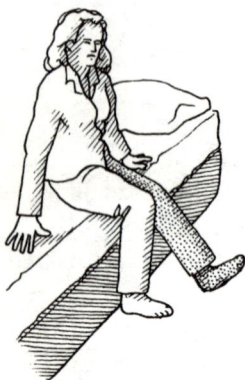

(c)

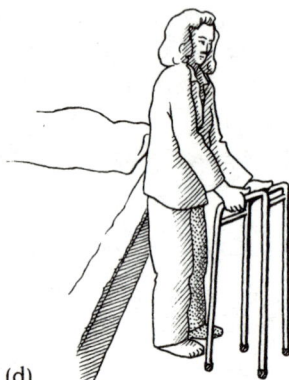

(d)

Getting out of bed. You should not get out of bed unaided after your operation until told it is safe for you to do so. *Keep your operated leg straight while you perform this manouevre*. (a) Sit up and swivel round on your bottom so that you are facing the side of the bed. (b) Sit on the edge of the bed and place the foot of your **un**operated leg on the floor. (c) Put your hands on the bed on either side of you and push down on them to help you to stand. Still keeping your operated leg straight, slide it back until your feet are side by side. When you are balanced, *and providing you do not feel dizzy or faint*, take hold of your walking frame, sticks or crutches. (The operated leg is shaded.)

GETTING INTO BED

To get into bed, stand near the bed with your back to it. Then lower your body until you are sitting on the edge of the bed, with your operated leg straight out in front of you. Swivel on your bottom and lift your **un**operated leg onto the bed first, followed by your operated one. You can then use your arms or a monkey pole (see p.44) to help you get into a comfortable position.

WALKING

Once you are up, and as long as you do not feel faint, the physiotherapist(s) will help you to walk a short distance with a walking frame. A couple of days or so later, you may be able to progress to walking with two crutches or two sticks. You will need crutches if your replacement joint is uncemented and therefore unable to bear your whole weight, but can probably use sticks if the joint is cemented and fully weight bearing.

Try to get into the habit as soon as possible of moving your *feet* to turn, taking small steps, rather than twisting your body and hip.

Possibly on the third or fourth post-operative day, the physiotherapist will show you how to do some exercises while standing to regain mobility and strength in your leg muscles. It is important to do these regularly and correctly. You should still continue to do the bed exercises described on page 64.

THE OCCUPATIONAL THERAPIST

Three or four days after your operation, when you are able to get out of bed and have regained some mobility, an occupational therapist will visit you on the ward to see how you are managing. Apart from making sure you are able to get out of bed, wash and dress yourself, the occupational therapist will help you to deal with any problems which may arise. He or she may visit you two or three times while you are in hospital to discuss any tasks you will have to do at home and to give you tips and advice to help you manage them more easily. Do ask about anything which worries you or which you are not sure you will be able to do. Also, if your relatives have any concerns, they can ask to talk to your occupational therapist, either when they visit you in hospital or by telephone.

WASHING AND DRESSING

If your wound is covered by a plastic film dressing, it may be possible for you to have showers before the stitches have been removed, although you may be advised to wait a couple of weeks to avoid the risk of infection being introduced through the wound before it has healed. Baths are best avoided for at least 10 to 12 weeks after your operation. Although boards are available which can be secured across a bath for you to sit on, they are quite difficult to use unless your arms are strong, and most only enable you to put your feet and lower legs in the bath water. There is also a risk of infection being introduced through the wound, the effects of which can be devastating.

Strip washes are the best way to keep clean until you are fully mobile and able to bend again. A nurse will wash your feet while you are in hospital and you will be given a stool to sit on at the washbasin for the first few days after your operation.

There are various aids available which you may find useful, for example long-handled shoehorns, hooked dressing sticks and stocking aids to help you put on your socks or stockings while you are unable to bend to reach your feet. The occupational therapist will explain their use to you, and you will be able to borrow any appropriate ones to take home for a few weeks.

USING THE TOILET

There will be special raised toilet seats in the hospital and a similar seat can be ordered for you to use at home if necessary.

(a) (b)

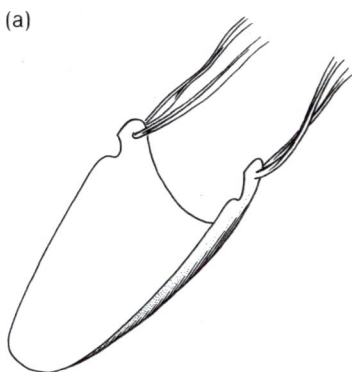

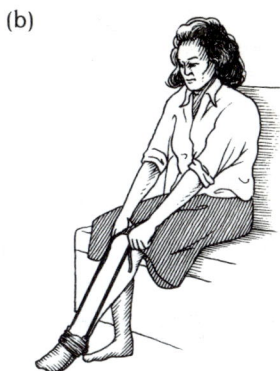

A stocking aid. Gather your sock or stocking over the end of the curved plastic mould and use the attached ribbons to swing it down to your foot. Slide your foot into the mould so that the sock or stocking is over your toes. Then gently pull on the ribbons to draw the sock or stocking up your leg until you can reach it without bending down.

To sit on the toilet, put one hand on the wall, washbasin or handrail for support. With your operated leg straight out in front of you, reach down to put your other hand onto the toilet seat behind you – without twisting your body. Lower yourself onto the seat, sliding your operated leg along the ground as you do so. To stand from the toilet, reverse this procedure.

STAIRS

By about the fifth or sixth post-operative day, the physiotherapist may help you to go up and down a flight of stairs using your crutches or sticks for support. Do not be disheartened if you are unable to master this technique immediately; it may take some practice. Even if your home is all on one level, you will need to be able to use stairs before you leave hospital so that you can step on and off kerbs and front-door steps etc.

Going up stairs

If the stairs have a handrail on one side only, put both your sticks or crutches in the opposite hand so that you can hold the handrail with the other. If there is a handrail on both sides of the stairs, still use only one, placing your sticks or crutches in the opposite hand. Place the foot of your **un**operated leg on the stair first, then the foot of your operated leg, and then your sticks or crutches. If there are no handrails, the sequence is still **un**operated leg, operated leg, sticks or crutches.

It is important to do this in the correct sequence so that you do not put all your weight on your operated leg and risk endangering your new hip.

Going down stairs

Whether you are using a handrail or coming down stairs without one, the sequence is the same. First place your walking sticks on the lower stair, then your operated leg, and then your **un**operated leg.

SITTING

You will not be allowed to sit in a chair until about the second post-operative day – later following revision surgery (see Chapter 11). The chairs in the hospital will be high and will have arms; you should have a similar chair, or one raised on blocks,

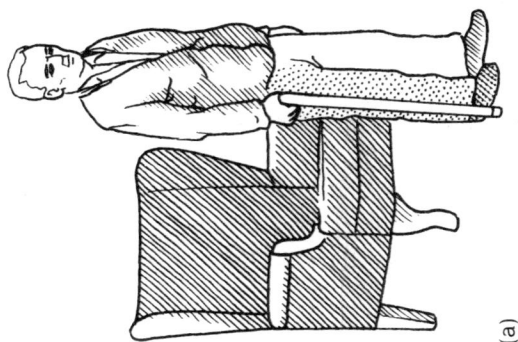

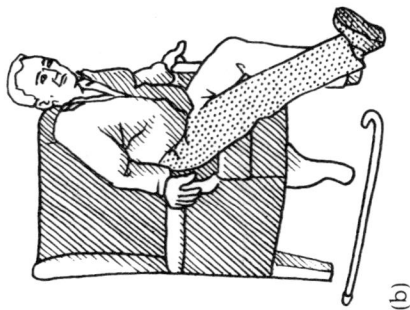

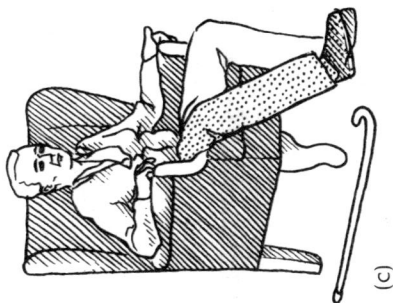

Sitting. (a) Stand in front of the chair with the backs of your legs touching it. (b) Place your hands on the arms of the chair, bend your **unoperated** leg and slide your operated leg out as you lower yourself on to the seat. (c) Keeping your operated leg straight, shuffle on your bottom to get comfortable. (The operated leg is shaded.)

at home. The physiotherapist will show you how to sit correctly to lessen hip flexion.

Once you have put your sticks or crutches safely to one side, stand with your back to the chair and the backs of your legs just touching its seat. Feel for the arms of the chair, one hand at a time, and hold onto them firmly. Do not twist your body around to look at the chair as you do this. Slide your operated leg straight out in front of you, bending your **un**operated leg at the knee as you sit down. Keep your hands on the arms of the chair and use them and your **un**operated leg to support your weight while you slide your bottom back onto the seat to get comfortable.

If you do have to sit on a chair which has no arms, stand with your back to its *side* and put one hand on the chair's back. Straighten your operated leg in front of you, bend your **un**operated leg at the knee, and lower yourself so that you can put your other hand on the chair seat. Once you are sitting, put both hands on the chair seat and swivel on your bottom, with your operated leg still straight, to face the right way and get comfortable.

SLEEPING

For about the first six months after your operation, you should only lie on your back with your thighs apart and your legs turned slightly outwards (abducted). While you are in hospital, a special abduction pillow may be placed between your legs to keep them in this position (see p.63). Once you are at home, two or three pillows between your legs will have the same effect.

You should avoid turning over in bed and should never lie on your operated side. After a few weeks you may be able to lie on your **un**operated side with your operated leg supported on pillows.

GOING HOME

Before you go home, the hospital staff must be satisfied that you will be able to manage. A medical social worker may visit you on the ward to discuss the help available through the social services, such as 'meals on wheels' or a home help. Do mention any potential problems to the medical social worker, occupational therapist or nursing staff *before* you leave hospital so that the social services can be alerted in good time if you are going to need assistance. If necessary, arrangements may be made to transfer you to a rehabilitation unit (see p.81) to continue physiotherapy and nursing care until you can manage alone at home.

When you are discharged from hospital, you may be given a letter to take to your family doctor or it may be sent directly to him or her by the hospital. This discharge letter will provide all the relevant information about your operation and any follow-up treatment you require, such as the removal of stitches. It should be delivered to your doctor's surgery as soon as possible.

GETTING INTO A CAR

You will probably go home in a car, and must therefore know how to get in and out of one. (Sports cars are not appropriate at this stage, nor is trying to get into the back of a car with only two doors.) It is helpful if the person taking you home from hospital can make the necessary adjustments to the position of the passenger seat before they collect you.

The car should be parked on level ground, leaving enough room between it and the pavement to allow you to step off the kerb and stand on the road. You can sit in the passenger seat, regardless of which hip has been operated on. The seat should be as far back as possible, with its back inclined at 45 degrees to upright. A plastic bin liner or carrier bag placed on the seat will help you to slide your bottom into position. The floor in front of the passenger seat should be free of bags and any other clutter.

With your back to the side of the car seat and your operated leg straight, lower yourself to sitting by bending your **un**operated leg. Once you are sitting down, slide your bottom over

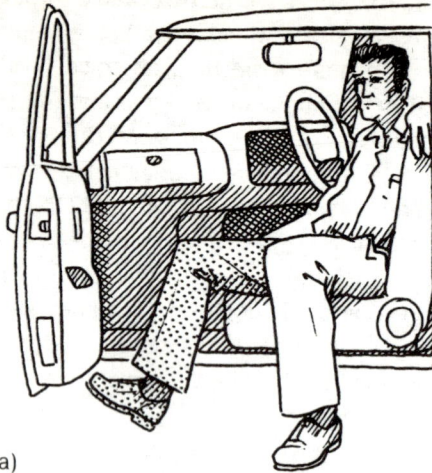

(a)

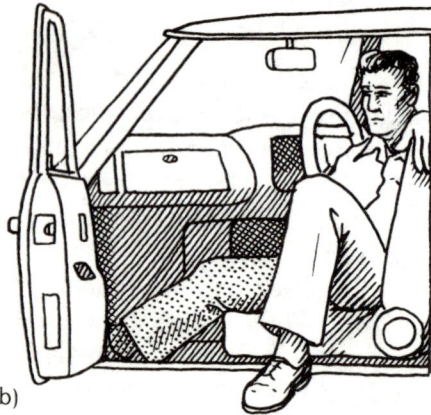

(b)

Getting into a car. *Keep your operated leg as straight as possible throughout this manouevre.* (a) Stand with your back to the side of the seat and lower yourself carefully onto its edge. (b) Slide your bottom well back onto the seat, leaning backwards slightly as you slowly swivel on your bottom to bring your operated leg into place in front of you. (The operated leg is shaded.)

towards the driver's seat as far as you can to leave yourself as much room as possible to manoeuvre. Swivel carefully on your bottom and bring your legs one at a time into the space in front of the seat – keeping your operated leg as straight as possible. It may help to lean back in the seat as you do this.

GETTING OUT OF A CAR

When getting out of the car, again slide your bottom towards the driver's seat and gently swing your legs out of the car, one at a time. Keep your operated leg out in front of you and put your weight onto your **un**operated leg as you raise yourself to standing.

As with all similar activities, it is important to take your time and move carefully, making sure that you keep your operated leg as straight as possible.

REHABILITATION UNITS

There are occasionally people who regain mobility slowly after hip replacement surgery, normally because they lack confidence. If medical staff think you will be unable to manage when the time comes for you to be discharged from hospital, you may be transferred to a rehabilitation unit for a few days before making the transition back home.

Rehabilitation units are staffed by nurses and normally have individual bedrooms, communal dining and sitting rooms and a kitchen where you can make drinks and snacks. Intensive efforts will be made by physiotherapists and occupational therapists to help you strengthen your leg muscles with exercises and to regain mobility and confidence by practising walking and various everyday activities.

However, these units are by no means universal, and this may not be an option in your area.

CHAPTER 9

After your operation: at home

By the time you leave hospital, you should be reasonably mobile and able to do most things for yourself at home, using any appropriate aids. However, your new hip will not be stable until three months after your operation, and strict adherence to your rehabilitation programme is essential during this time. You will be given any necessary advice before you are discharged, including how and when to use your walking aids.

Although the risk of dislocating your new hip joint is greatest in the weeks immediately following your operation, it will remain for life, and you should always take care to avoid awkward positioning of your operated leg and strenuous sporting activities.

DAILY ACTIVITIES

It is important that you keep reasonably active, without overdoing it. You should avoid standing for long periods and, if you do have to do jobs such as ironing or preparing meals, make sure you do them sitting down. You will need someone to do your shopping and heavy housework for a couple of weeks at least. The effort and care you put into your rehabilitation programme will ensure you make good and steady progress and do not risk dislocating your new hip or setting your recovery back in any other way.

If you have any specific mobility problems, you may be told

to do special exercises or hydrotherapy for some time after your operation or you may continue to see a physiotherapist at regular out-patient appointments to deal with a particular difficulty. Otherwise, remembering the special precautions mentioned on page 70 and continuing the exercises you have been shown should help you to resume the level of activity appropriate for your lifestyle.

There will be restrictions on what you can do for two or three months after your operation.

* *Walking*. Walking is very good exercise – in moderation – but you should avoid walking on uneven or slippery surfaces.

* *Sitting*. Avoid sitting on low or very soft chairs and, whenever possible, on chairs without arms. If necessary, use chair blocks, available on loan from the hospital.

* *Washing and dressing*. Unless you have a bath board and are confident that your arms are strong enough to support you while getting on and off it, continue to strip wash rather than bathing for the first few weeks. You can have showers if your stitches have been removed or your wound is covered with a waterproof dressing. However, if you have a shower attachment over your bath, you may need to sit on a bath board while showering.

  Do not bend to cut your toenails, put on your shoes and socks etc. for the first 12 weeks or so after your operation or until advised that it is safe to do so. Thereafter, *always* take care not to bend too far when washing or dressing to avoid dislocating your hip. Before you leave hospital, you will be given any dressing aids which may be useful – such as a sock or stocking aid, a dressing hook or long-handled shoehorn. If possible, wear slip-on shoes to avoid having to tie laces.

* *Using the toilet*. You will need some support as you get on and off the toilet seat, and if there is no wall or washbasin near

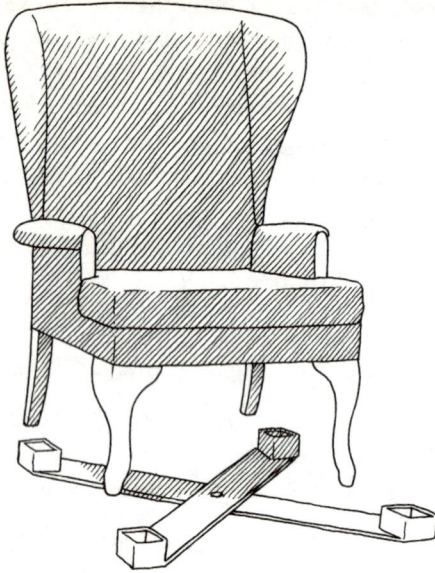

Chair blocks. Blocks like these can be placed under the legs of a chair to raise it by about 5 cm (2 inches). Tighten the wing nuts on each block so that the chair legs are gripped securely.

your toilet at home, you may be given a raised toilet seat with handrails attached or it may be suggested that a handrail is fixed to a nearby wall. The occupational therapist will discuss these options with you.

* *Driving*. It may be possible to resume driving after your first follow-up appointment, but you should not drive until your consultant says it is safe to do so. If you have a very small car or a sports car, you may have to wait until stability and a good range of motion have been achieved.

Driving should be avoided for three or four months following revision surgery.

* *Exercise and sport.* You will have been told by the physiotherapist at the hospital how to do the exercises necessary to
restore the muscle strength and mobility to your leg and hip
joint. Specific exercises have not been included here as it is
important that you only do the ones you have been shown.

Gentle exercise is important, but if you attend an exercise
class, you should tell your instructor you have had a hip
replacement operation. Supervised exercise in a swimming
pool can be helpful during the first few post-operative
months, gradually progressing to gentle swimming as
mobility and comfort return. You should not do breast
stroke for at least three months after your operation
because of the leg movements involved.

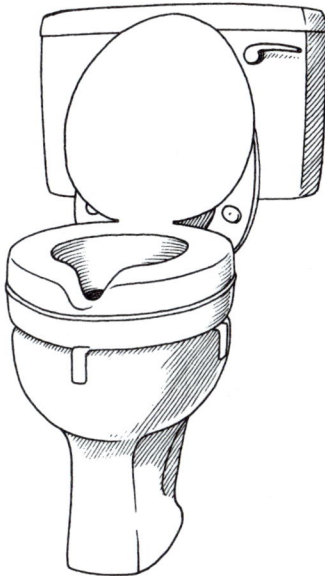

A raised toilet seat. This type of raised seat has three brackets to
secure it to the toilet.

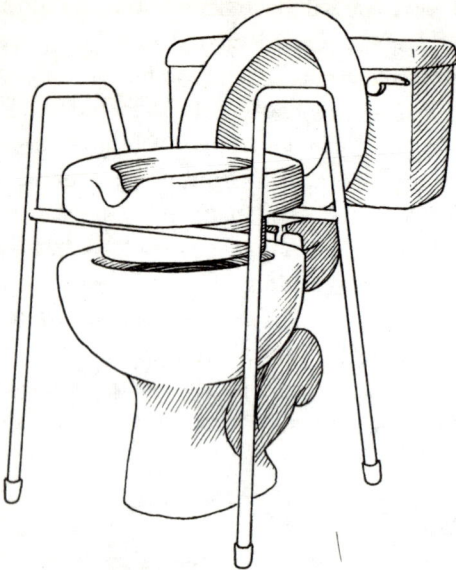

A raised toilet seat with handrails. The seat is secured to the rim of the toilet by catches. The telescopic legs on the frame can be adjusted so that the handrails are appropriate for your height.

If you wish to ride a bicycle, you should be able to do so after about three months, when you are able to bend your leg sufficiently. You should also be able to do gardening after the first few post-operative weeks, but always avoid flexing your operated leg too much or putting it in an awkward position. Ballroom dancing should be possible as soon as you feel confident enough to do it.

Vigorous sports are never appropriate after hip replacement surgery.

* *Sexual intercourse.* You will probably be able to resume sexual intercourse about six weeks after your operation. When movement has become pain free, you can lie on the side of your **un**operated leg, with a pillow to support your operated

leg. After a few months you will be able to have sexual intercourse while lying on your back or on top of your partner, but you should continue to avoid bending your operated leg beyond an angle of 90 degrees.

* *Driving and insurance.* It has been known for someone to be the blameless driver in a road accident several weeks after hip replacement surgery, only to find that their own insurance was invalid because they had not notified their insurance company of their operation. It is therefore a good idea to check your car insurance policy before you start driving again and, if necessary, to write to your insurance company to tell them you have had hip replacement surgery.

Apart from following all the advice and instructions concerning your rehabilitation programme, it is important to use your commonsense at all times and to avoid doing anything which could endanger your new hip during the three months it takes to stabilise.

FOLLOW-UP APPOINTMENTS

You will be given an out-patient appointment about six to eight weeks after your operation, during which your hip will be examined and an X-ray taken of it.

Another follow-up appointment will probably be made for about six months after surgery, during which further X-rays will be taken and you will be assessed by the surgeon and a physiotherapist. By this time, you are likely to be able to walk without limping, and to have regained enough mobility and muscle strength to allow you to resume your normal daily activities.

During the weeks following your hip replacement operation, do make a note of any questions you wish to ask and take it with you to your follow-up appointment.

CHAPTER 10

Possible post-operative complications

There are some general complications which can occur after any type of operation, and some which are specifically related to hip replacement surgery. Most complications are minor, but occasionally more serious ones arise and it is important to be aware of these and to seek medical attention if you are at all concerned. Apart from the complications which may develop within hours or days of surgery, there are others which may not become apparent for months, or even years.

GENERAL COMPLICATIONS

The general complications described here can occur in some form after any operation and, where necessary, precautions will be taken to reduce their risk.

Chest infection

Chest infection is possible following general anaesthesia, and it is particularly common in smokers. Deep breathing is important post-operatively to keep the lungs clear but, if necessary, a physiotherapist will visit you on the ward to advise you about appropriate exercises.

Pyrexia

Pyrexia is fever. It can develop in the first 24 to 72 hours after surgery but if it persists, its cause will have to be investigated. Amongst other causes, pyrexia can be due to a chest or wound infection or to deep vein thrombosis (see below).

Thrombosis and embolism

Deep vein thrombosis occurs when a blood clot forms in one of the deep veins of the body – usually in the calf veins of the legs. Its potential danger is associated with the risk of the blood clot breaking away and lodging, for example, in the lungs, causing a pulmonary embolism.

It has been estimated, in both the UK and the USA, that approximately 50 per cent of people undergoing surgery to the lower extremities develop deep vein thrombosis. This relatively high incidence is partly due to the fact that surgery involving bone releases a substance called **thromboplastin** which plays a role in the natural process of the formation of blood clots. Surgery can also cause distension of the valve cusps which control the flow of blood through the blood vessels, thus leading to the pooling of blood (known as **stasis**) within the veins of the leg.

Precautions such as the wearing of anti-embolism stockings, a course of low-dose heparin or warfarin injections to thin the blood and help prevent clotting, exercises and, importantly, becoming mobile as soon as possible after your operation should help to prevent thrombosis.

Thrombosis in the *calf* rarely leads to pulmonary embolism (which is associated more commonly with thrombosis in the *thigh*), but it is important to be aware of its signs and symptoms and to seek medical attention immediately. A blood clot may be symptomless, possibly developing 48 hours or more after surgery, or it may give rise to local tenderness, swelling, fever and pain. Treatment will be necessary to avoid further complications; pulmonary embolism is more difficult to treat. Treatment of a thrombus in the calf usually involves bed rest and elevation of the affected leg, with or without the use of higher doses of intravenous heparin or warfarin. Deep vein thrombosis in the thigh will need to be very carefully monitored in hospital and higher-dose heparin or warfarin injections will sometimes have to be continued for three months or longer.

Infection

Infection is always a risk when materials are implanted into the body. Operating theatres in which hip replacement surgery takes place are therefore fitted with special ventilation systems to clean the air. In some centres, operating staff also wear body suits, similar in appearance to space suits. Antibiotics are normally given for 24 hours before and after surgery, and sometimes for longer. For people at high risk (and often routinely), the cement used to fix an implant is sometimes impregnated with antibiotic which leaches out over the ensuing weeks to provide some additional protection against the multiplication of bacteria in the immediate area.

Sepsis

Sepsis is infection caused by pus-producing organisms. Once present, it is difficult to cure. Deep sepsis is catastrophic and usually leads to joint failure, with the need to remove the replacement hip joint to control the infection. A new hip may either be inserted at the time of removal of the old one or 6 to 12 weeks later. Sepsis may cause long-term disability.

Despite the precautions taken, the main cause of sepsis is contamination of the wound during surgery, either with airborne bacteria or with bacteria transferred from the patient's skin. It may also occur after surgery if bacteria are transferred to the operation site via the blood or lymph from a urinary tract infection, skin break or abscess etc. Therefore, the skin over the operating site is always examined carefully before surgery and if there are any skin breaks or abrasions, the operation may be postponed until they have healed. Surgery may also be postponed if, when your mouth is examined pre-operatively, you are found to require dental repairs. A sample of your urine will be analysed before your operation to detect the presence of any urinary tract infection. Once in the operating theatre, the operation site will be cleaned with an antiseptic solution and your body will be covered with sterile drapes.

The risk of post-operative sepsis may also be increased if there is a delay in wound healing.

Although the incidence of sepsis immediately after hip operations is declining, due to the precautionary measures described, it does still occur, even a year or more after surgery and sometimes because an infection has remained latent since a previous operation or injury.

People at increased risk of sepsis include those with auto-immune diseases, rheumatoid arthritis, systemic lupus erythematosus or diabetes, as well as those who are corticosteroid dependent. Its incidence doubles following revision surgery.

Wound infection

Infection sometimes occurs in the wound following any operation. Primary wound healing is important and if your wound continues to ooze a bloody discharge, you may be started on a course of antibiotics and kept in hospital until it has completely healed. Occasionally, germs collect around the stitches, some of which may have to be removed to allow an infected discharge to escape.

It is possible, weeks or months after surgery, for an infection to arise if foreign bodies such as suture material have been left within the wound. Infection can also develop in a wound as a result of spread of infective organisms from elsewhere in the body, when it is known as **metastatic infection**.

You should seek medical attention if you have the following

signs: pain, swelling, heat and redness around the wound, possibly with leakage of pus or infected fluid, and a high body temperature.

Nerve damage

The small nerves supplying the skin over the operation site are usually damaged when an incision is made during surgery, occasionally causing a small area around the wound to remain permanently numb. Although the size of the area of numbness will decrease with time, the sensation may never return completely.

Neuroma
Very rarely, small, painful, tender areas form in part of the scar, which may be due to a swelling of the cut nerve ends known as a neuroma. Nerve damage may lead to pain in the wound which will be relieved temporarily by the injection of local anaesthetic. Continued pain may respond to steroid injection. Only rarely is surgery needed to remove a painful nodule.

Nerve palsy
The nerve damage which can occur during an operation can cause loss of sensation, and possibly power, which may last for days or months but which will eventually recover to a greater or lesser extent as the nerves regenerate. However, depending on the damage to the nerves, they may never fully repair themselves and loss of function of the affected part – known as nerve palsy – can develop. Nerve palsy is more common in women (for reasons which are not fully understood) and following revision surgery.

Bleeding and bruising

There is often a certain amount of oozing of blood or fluid from the wound, but this is unlikely to be heavy. If it continues, and particularly if leakage occurs through the wound dressing and soils your clothes, medical advice should be sought. On rare occasions, a second operation is required to tie off or cauterise a bleeding blood vessel which was overlooked or which has started to bleed again post-operatively.

Occasionally, blood which does not escape through the edges of the wound may give rise to severe bruising, possibly several days after surgery. Although the sight of the bruise may be distressing, treatment is only seldom required to release the blood which has accumulated under the skin.

Haematoma

In rare cases, a haematoma may develop. A haematoma is a swelling which is full of blood and is caused by a blood vessel either continuing to bleed or re-opening after surgery, or by a collection of blood oozing into a space created during surgery. It can sometimes result from a disturbance of the normal blood-clotting mechanisms of the body, for example caused by anticoagulants such as heparin. There are also inherited bleeding disorders, such as haemophilia, which cause a similar disturbance of the blood-clotting mechanism, but these conditions will be taken into account before any operation is considered.

Haematoma development is accompanied by pain, the formation of a hard swelling, and possibly a reddish purple discoloration of the skin. Bruising may appear around the wound or at some distance from it over the next few days. A raised body temperature may result from the haematoma itself or from infection in the wound (see above).

If you think a haematoma is forming or has formed once you have left hospital, you should contact your family doctor or consultant for advice. The blood is likely to be reabsorbed spontaneously within three or four weeks without the need for any treatment, but if heavy bleeding continues, with increased pain and swelling, you may need surgery to close off the blood vessel which is causing it. Your doctor may also wish to do specialised blood tests to check that your blood-clotting factors are normal.

COMPLICATIONS OF HIP REPLACEMENT SURGERY

Apart from the general complications of surgery described above, the following are specifically related to hip replacement surgery. For most of them, the risk is increased following revision surgery.

Dislocation

Dislocation of the hip joint is not a common complication, although its risk is increased after revision surgery. It involves complete displacement of the head of the femur from its normal position in the acetabulum. **Subluxation** (incomplete dislocation) is also possible: there may be an audible click as the head of the femur moves onto the rim of the acetabulum and again as it re-enters the socket of the joint.

Most dislocations occur within two months of hip replacement surgery, although they occasionally arise five or more years later. They are most common in people with post-traumatic osteoarthritis, congenital hip dysplasia, neuromuscular diseases or muscle weakness, although the cause is often unknown. A dislocated joint will cause the affected leg to be held in an abnormal position and to appear short in relation to the other leg. Attempts to rotate the leg at the hip joint are painful. It is important always to follow the advice given on page 70 to help reduce the risk of dislocation.

A dislocated hip may be reduced while you are under sedation or under general anaesthesia in an operating theatre.

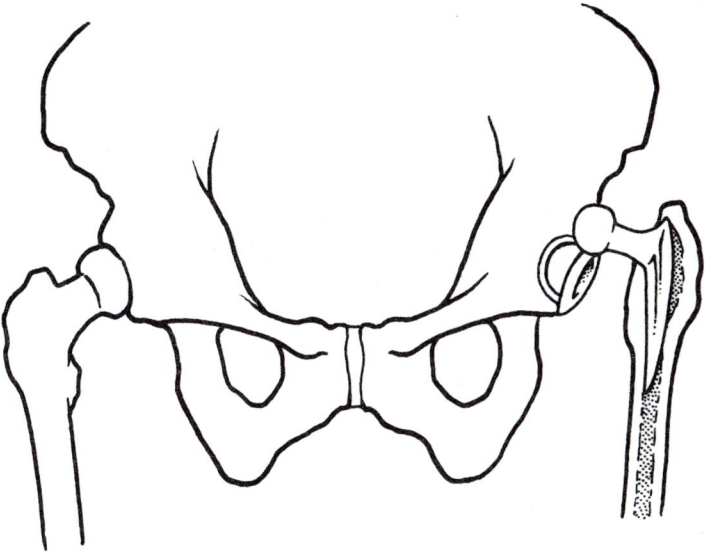

Dislocation. The head of the femoral component has become dislodged from its correct position within the socket formed by the acetabular component.

Heterotopic bone formation

Heterotopic bone formation is the development of bone in an area of the body in which it is not normally produced. It occurs occasionally follow hip replacement surgery and, when severe, mobility may be reduced or even lost completely. Bone may form within the soft tissues around the hip, or it may protrude in spurs from the pelvis or the end of the femur.

Preventative measures – for example low doses of radiation given post-operatively – are necessary for people considered at high risk, such as those with previous heterotopic bone formation, trauma, osteoarthritis or ankylosing spondylitis. Non-steroidal anti-inflammatory drugs (NSAIDs), commonly indomethacin or ibuprofen, may be given prophylactically. Although these drugs may inhibit abnormal ossification, they can also reduce the *desired* ingrowth of bone into porous-coated prostheses and are therefore not given post-operatively to people with cementless prostheses coated, for example, with cobalt chrome beads. They are also inappropriate for people taking warfarin to reduce the risk of blood clots as the two drugs together can induce heavy bleeding from the gastrointestinal tract.

If heterotopic bone formation occurs and interferes with mobility, the abnormal bone may be removed surgically once it has fully matured, usually six months or more after the replacement hip operation.

Aseptic loosening

In the past, it was not unusual for a component of a replacement hip joint to fail, but this risk has been much reduced by the use of stronger modern alloys and improved design.

Aseptic loosening (i.e. loosening of a component caused by something other than infection) is now the most common cause of component failure. It may be the result of a less-than-perfect surgical technique, poor quality or quantity of the bone to which the prosthesis has been attached, excessive body weight, or inappropriate or excessive activity, all of which may lead to absorption and breakdown of the bone (osteolysis).

Failure may occur between the cement or porous coating and the bone, or between the prosthesis and the cement. Where possible, aseptic loosening is treated by revising the hip replacement.

Foreign body reaction

A problem with plastic components is that they may wear, producing debris which can cause a foreign body reaction. Degradation of cement can lead to resorption of the bone stock and thus component loosening (see above). The generation of debris may produce osteolysis in the acetabulum or the femur which is usually associated with pain and loosening of the implant.

Fracture

Very rarely, a hip replacement operation may fail due to fracture of the pelvis or acetabulum. Fracture of the femur around an implanted stem is a slightly less rare, but serious, complication. Sometimes loosening of an implant, associated with osteolysis (see above), weakens the bone stock and may predispose to fracture. Fractures may also result from post-operative injury or trauma, bone disorders or osteoporosis (see p.8), and are more common after revision surgery. They may occur *during* surgery if the operation is difficult to perform or the bone is weakened for any reason.

CHAPTER 11

Revision surgery

Sometimes hip replacements fail, possibly (but not commonly) as a result of infection or some other complication, or because the components have worn with the passage of time. If failure occurs, revision surgery will be necessary to remove the primary hip replacement and implant new components. Although it is possible to repeat revision surgery – in theory at least, as many times as necessary – the results do tend to become progressively less good. The amount of scar tissue produced after any type of surgery increases with each successive operation. Following even a first revision operation, the muscles of the leg may not work as well as after a primary hip replacement, and occasional aches in the legs are relatively common. In many respects, the details of the preparation for and recovery from revision surgery are similar to those of primary hip replacement, but some aspects of the two types of operation do differ.

BEFORE THE OPERATION

The pre-operative tests done prior to revision surgery are basically the same as those described in Chapter 2. Before revision surgery is undertaken it is very important that any existing infection is detected and treated. Infection present in the primary hip replacement could recur in the revised hip, possibly causing the components to loosen. Therefore, you are likely to have blood tests, isotope scans and **aspiration** to detect infective organisms in your hip joint or elsewhere in your body. Aspiration may be done under a local or general anaesthetic and involves the insertion of a needle into the hip to remove a sample of fluid from it, which is then examined for the presence of bacteria.

THE OPERATIONS

If no infection is detected, it is often possible to remove the primary hip replacement and insert the new components in a single operation. However, if infection is present, a two-stage revision may be performed. This involves doing an excision arthroplasty (see p.10) to remove the primary hip replacement and then treating the infection to eradicate it completely before a second operation is done to insert the new components. The period between the two operations may be about six weeks or longer. It is usually possible to walk with the aid of two crutches or walking sticks in the absence of a hip joint while awaiting the second operation.

Revision surgery is normally done under a general anaesthetic, and often takes three to four hours or longer. The procedure used depends largely on the difficulty encountered in retrieving the components of the primary hip replacement. Sometimes, over the years, the acetabular component becomes loose and protrudes inwards towards the bladder. If this happens, it may have to be retrieved from inside the pelvis. Locating and removing the acetabular component can thus be technically difficult, as can the removal of the cement of a cement-fixed prosthesis. Usually, a number of small, metal, chisel-like instruments called **osteotomes** are used to chip away the cement from the hole in the femur into which the femoral component was inserted. Occasionally, a cutting drill is required or, more rarely, lasers or ultrasound.

The second part of a one-stage revision, or the second operation of a two-stage revision, involves **reconstruction** of the existing bone and insertion of the new components. When a primary hip replacement has been in place for several years, there may be quite significant loss of bone stock, which means the bones will be weak. Therefore, the bone must first be reconstructed by grafting to avoid premature failure of the components.

Reconstruction can be done by means of an **autograft**, using bone taken from the pelvis of the patient, although the amount of bone available for this type of graft is often limited. Therefore, in countries with bone banks, it is more common to use **allograft**, which is bone from another individual. Occasionally, a **xenograft** is done with bone from an animal, or artificial manufactured **bone substitute** is used. The two latter types of graft are less common and tend to be less successful.

Although it may be possible to insert the same type of components as those used for the primary hip replacement, there are special femoral components with longer stems or broader bodies designed specifically for revision surgery. The risk of loosening and protrusion of the acetabular component can be avoided by inserting retaining metal mesh or by attaching metal reinforcement rings to the outer wall of the pelvis by means of screws or hooks to fill in any bone defects.

AFTER THE OPERATION

The post-operative care and rehabilitation following revision surgery are similar to those of a primary operation, and you will probably be in hospital for about the same length of time (up to two weeks). You may need to use crutches for longer and may have to wear a hip brace to hold your new joint in position while the tissues heal.

CHAPTER 12

Private care

In countries such as Britain where there is a state health service, there are various reasons why people choose to have their operations done privately. They may have private health insurance, or be covered by a private health scheme run by the company for which they work, or they may be able to pay for private care themselves. Whatever your situation, you will not find that the *standard* of medical care you receive in a private hospital is any different from that available on the National Health Service. But you may prefer the privacy of a private hospital, or you may find it more convenient to be able to enter hospital for your operation at the time of your choice. The waiting time for hip surgery varies around the country, and can be anything from a couple of months to a year or more. For anyone suffering pain and severe restrictions to their lifestyle due to reduced mobility, private treatment may therefore be an attractive option — although quite a costly one.

If you have an operation in an NHS hospital, you may not see the consultant at all, being examined and treated by different doctors in the consultant's firm. At a private hospital, you will receive personal care from the consultant throughout your stay. The facilities at a private hospital are likely to be similar to those of a good hotel, and will certainly include a private bathroom.

The information given in other chapters in this book is equally relevant whichever system you choose. This chapter explains the practicalities of obtaining private health care and deals with the differences between the two systems.

PRIVATE HEALTH INSURANCE

If you work for a company which has a private health insurance scheme, your Company Secretary will be able to give you details, and should be able to tell you if the company insurance covers you for your operation.

If you have your own private health insurance, someone at the insurance company will be able to tell you exactly what is covered by your particular policy if this is not clear from the literature you already have. It is always worth checking anyway, and asking for *written* confirmation. Do not be afraid to keep asking questions until you are certain you know exactly which costs you will be responsible for paying yourself. For example, does your insurance cover all follow-up appointments?

There are different levels of health insurance, and you need to make sure you know which costs are included. Most private hospitals have an administration officer who will check your policy for you if you are in any doubt. The staff at the hospital are likely to be very helpful and will try to sort out any problems and queries you have. But do read your policy carefully, as well as any information sent to you by the hospital, as unexpected charges, such as consultants' fees which may not be covered, could add up to quite a lot of money.

With some types of private health insurance, you will need to ask your family doctor to fill in a form stating that your operation is necessary and cannot be done in an NHS hospital within a certain time period due to long waiting lists. You will have to pay your doctor for this service, which will cost a few pounds. This money is not redeemable from your insurers.

FIXED PRICE CARE

If you think you may be able to pay to have your operation done privately, the Bookings Manager at a private hospital can give you an idea of the cost involved. Some private hospitals run a service known as Fixed Price Care: a price can be quoted to you before you enter hospital which covers your operation and a variety of other hospitalisation costs. You should always ask to have the quotation in writing *before* you enter hospital, with a written note of everything it includes. At some hospitals, the fixed price will include accommodation, nursing, meals, drugs, dressings, operating theatre fees, X-rays etc.; at others only some of these are included. Once you have a quotation, you should not have to worry about any hidden costs for which you had not accounted. However, the price quoted to you may not include the fees of the consultant surgeon or anaesthetist, and you may have to ask your consultant for a note of these.

With Fixed Price Care, all the hospitalisation costs included by that particular hospital are covered should a complication arise which is directly related to your hip problem or the surgery to treat it and which necessitates you staying longer in hospital, usually up to a maximum of 28 days. Again, consultants' fees will probably be extra. However, if you develop some problem while in hospital which is unrelated to your original hip problem, the price you have been quoted will not cover treatment to deal with this. At some hospitals, the quoted price will also include your treatment should you have to be re-admitted due to a complication related to your original operation and arising within a limited period of time after your discharge.

The only extra charges you will have to pay to the hospital will probably include those for telephone calls, any alcohol if you have this with your meals, food provided for your visitors, personal laundry done by the hospital and any similar items such as you would have to pay for in a hotel. It is usually possible for a visitor to eat meals with you in your room, and for tea and snacks to be ordered for visitors during the day. (You will also have to pay these extra charges before you leave the hospital if you are being treated under private health insurance.)

It is important therefore that you ask in advance for *written* confirmation of the price you will have to pay for your stay in hospital and what is included in the quotation. If the hospital does not have a Fixed Price Care or similar system, make sure that all possible costs are listed.

ARRANGING THE OPERATION

As for treatment under the NHS, you will have to be referred to see a consultant privately by your family doctor. Most doctors have contacts with particular consultants (and private hospitals) to whom they tend to refer patients. If there is a private hospital you particularly want to go to, or a consultant you have some reason to prefer, you can ask your family doctor to make an appointment for you.

After your visit to your doctor, you are unlikely to have to wait longer than a week or two before you see the consultant at an out-patient appointment. Your appointment may be at the private hospital where your operation is to be carried out, at an NHS hospital which has private wards, or at the consultant's private consulting rooms. Once the decision has been made to go ahead with surgery, you will probably be able to enter hospital at your convenience within another week or two.

You will receive confirmation of the date of your operation from the Bookings Manager of the hospital you are to attend. You may also be sent leaflets and any further relevant details about your admission to hospital. Do read these carefully, as knowing how a particular hospital organises things will help you to be prepared when you arrive for your operation. You will also be sent a **pre-admission form** to fill in and take with you when you are admitted.

If your operation is being paid for by insurance, you will be asked to take a completed insurance form with you when you are admitted to hospital. You should have been given some of these forms when you first took out your policy, but your insurance company will be able to supply the correct one if you have any problems. If you are covered by company insurance, the form will probably be filled in and given to you by your Company Secretary.

ADMISSION AND DISCHARGE

When you arrive at the hospital, the receptionist will contact the admissions department, and a ward receptionist will come to collect you. If you are paying for your treatment yourself, you will probably be asked to pay your bill in advance at this stage if you have not already done so. Otherwise, you will be asked for your completed insurance form. The ward receptionist will take you to your room – probably a single or double room – and show you the facilities available there. You are likely to have a private bathroom, a television, and a telephone by your bed. The ward receptionist will explain hospital procedures to you, and will leave you to settle in.

A member of the nursing staff will then come to make a note of your medical details, in much the same way as described in Chapter 5. The main difference you are likely to notice if you have been treated in an NHS hospital before, is that this time there is much less waiting for all the routine hospital procedures to be dealt with. The nurse to patient ratio is higher in private hospitals and so someone is usually available to deal with the pre-operative procedures quite quickly.

Your consultant will take charge of your medical care throughout your stay, will visit you before the operation, perform the operation (with the assistance of the anaesthetist and the operating staff), and visit you again when you are back in your own room. Trainees – whether doctors or nurses – do not work in private hospitals. The consultants are responsible for their own patients and supervise their care themselves. Most private hospitals now have resident medical officers – fully qualified, registered doctors who are available 24 hours a day to deal with any emergencies which may arise.

When the time for your operation approaches, a porter and nurse will take you from your room to the anaesthetic room. In many private hospitals, you will not be moved from your bed onto a trolley until you have been anaesthetised; the bed itself will be wheeled from your room. Similarly, you will be transferred back from the trolley to your own bed in the recovery room while you are still asleep. You therefore go to sleep and wake up in your own hospital bed.

Your operation will be performed in the same way as described in Chapter 7. When you are fully awake, you will be taken back to your room to rest.

When you are ready to be discharged from hospital, the ward receptionist will ask you to pay any outstanding charges not covered by the hospitalisation charge, and you will be given any medical items you may need from the hospital pharmacy.

SUMMARY

The main aim of the staff of any private hospital is the same as that in an NHS hospital – to make your stay as pleasant and as comfortable as possible. Because the staffing ratio is higher in private hospitals, more emphasis can be placed on privacy and comfort.

The consultant surgeons and anaesthetists almost always work in an NHS hospital as well as in a private hospital, so you will receive the same expertise and skill under both systems. However, in an NHS hospital you may not actually be operated on by the consultant surgeon who heads the surgical team and, indeed, you may not see the consultant at all during your stay.

Private hospitals arrange their operating lists differently from NHS hospitals. The latter have 'sessional bookings' for their operating theatres. This means a particular day is set aside at regular intervals for a specialist in one type of surgery to perform operations. In private hospitals, the consultants can book the use of an operating theatre (and the assistance of the staff who work in it) on more or less any day, at any time that suits them. Therefore, your operation can take place privately at a time that is convenient to you and your consultant.

It is also possible, even if you are already on an NHS waiting list, to tell your family doctor or consultant at any time that you would like to change to private care. If the consultant you have already seen under the NHS does not have a private practice, you can ask to be put in touch with one who *can* see you privately.

There are several reasons why, if they can, some people choose to have their operations done privately, either paid for by private health insurance or from their own pockets. Some find it more convenient to be able to have a say in when their operation is to take place, particularly if this means avoiding a wait of several months or more. Some simply prefer the smaller, more intimate setting they are likely to find in a private hospital. As private hospitals rarely deal with accidents and emergency treatment (the operations carried out in them normally being planned at least a day or two in advance), they do not have the bustle of an NHS hospital which has to deal with emergency admissions as well as the routine admissions for non-emergency operations.

Questions and answers

The answers to most of the questions below can be found elsewhere in the book. However, you may find this section helpful in compiling your own list to ask your family doctor or consultant. The answers given here are general and the specific information you are given may be slightly different, according to what happens at your particular hospital.

Always ask your family doctor, the hospital doctor who is in charge of your care, or a nurse whenever you do not understand something. No question is too trivial, particularly if it concerns something that is worrying you.

1. *I am 55 and for many years have been a keen squash player. Over the last few years I have suffered from a stiff and painful hip joint which has gradually deteriorated to the point where I can no longer play squash at all, or any other active sport. Would a hip replacement operation enable me to take up squash again?*

Hip replacement operations are done to relieve pain, improve mobility and enable people to lead reasonably active lives again. However, taking part in any vigorous sports after hip replacement surgery will not only increase the risk of dislocation, but will also reduce the life of the implanted joint and should therefore be avoided.

A hip replacement done at your relatively young age is likely to need revision – possibly after 10 or 15 years – and therefore might not be thought appropriate for the time being. On the other hand, if the disability and pain you are suffering can no longer be eased by drugs and physiotherapy, and your normal daily life is significantly restricted, an oper- ation may be considered despite your age. But whether or not you have an operation, you will have to accept that squash and other energetic sports will no longer be possible.

Do talk to your family doctor about your problems and about the treatment options available for you.

2. How long will it be until I am able to walk without a stick and resume all my normal activities after my hip replacement operation?

People make progress at different rates after hip replacement surgery, depending on various factors such as their age, general health and level of fitness and how quickly their confidence returns. If all goes well, you could be walking unaided and be able to do most everyday activities after two to three months. However, although the risk of dislocation reduces after a few weeks, you will always have to take a few precautions such as avoiding crossing your legs, positioning them awkwardly or raising your operated leg too high.

3. Both my hip joints have been damaged by osteoarthritis and I am becoming increasing disabled by pain and stiffness. Would I be able to have both hips replaced at the same time?

Bilateral hip replacement is not usually carried out at a single operation, for several reasons. It is much more difficult to regain mobility post-operatively if you do not have a 'good' leg to support you. It is also advisable to make sure that surgery is successful on one leg before attempting an operation on the other, and you will need time to recover fully from your first operation and to regain mobility before your second hip is replaced. However, if it is thought that your rehabilitation following replacement of one hip would be severely restricted by pain and deformity in the other, your consultant may consider replacing both hip joints at the same time.

Your family doctor or orthopaedic consultant will be able to advise you and, if a decision is made to do two separate operations, should be able to tell you approximately how long it is likely to be before you could have your second hip replaced.

4. I am on a waiting list for hip replacement surgery, but understand it may be several months before it takes place. Is it too late to find out about having the operation done privately and, if not, who should I ask about this?

You can ask your family doctor at any time to refer you to a consultant privately and you should be able to remain on the NHS waiting list until you have made your decision. You will have to pay your doctor a small fee for this referral.

Do make sure you ask the consultant and the private hospital for a written note of the costs involved before you opt to have your operation done privately as these are likely to amount to several thousand pounds.

5. My father is due to have a hip replacement operation next month and I had planned for him to stay with me when he comes out of hospital. However, due to an unexpected work commitment, it now looks as though this will not be possible. What can I do to make sure he is not sent home alone when he is discharged from hospital, and is there any practical help which would be available for him?

There are various services which could be arranged for your father, such as 'meals on wheels' and a home help and, if necessary, someone can visit him daily at specific times to help him dress etc. You should contact the Department of Social Services in the area in which your father lives and explain the situation to them. If he has already had a pre-operative assessment, you should also contact the hospital ward to which he is to be admitted and the occupational therapist at the hospital to tell them of the change of plan so that new arrangements can be made for him in good time.

However, do be reassured that your father will not be discharged from hospital until medical staff are satisfied that he will be able to manage at home, either alone or with the assistance mentioned above. If necessary, arrangements may be made for him to be transferred to a rehabilitation unit when he is discharged from hospital so that he can continue to do exercises and practise various household chores under supervision until he is ready to manage at home.

6. When I had my hip replaced six weeks ago, I was told I would need to use a walking stick for at least two months. As I feel fine already and can walk quite easily without support, is it all right stop using my stick now?

You should continue to use your walking stick as advised, at least until your follow-up appointment. However well you may feel, the muscles and other tissues in your leg need time to heal properly and your new hip joint needs to stabilise before you walk unaided and this process takes three months. It is not worth risking a fall and the good progress you have already made by putting too much strain on your new hip too soon.

7. I had a hip replacement operation about five months ago. Recently, my hip seemed to 'click' and was painful for a short time, although it seems all right now. What could this have been and is it likely to happen again?

Although there are several, less important circumstances which may produce a click, it is possible that the sound you heard was the implanted head of your thigh bone slipping out of its position in the socket in your pelvic bone and then falling back into place. This is a partial dislocation known as subluxation and there is no way of telling if it will happen again. Always be careful to avoid twisting your hip or lifting your leg too high as these movements could cause the joint to dislocate. If you are concerned or if it does occur again, ask your doctor's advice.

8. I am 83 and have had a painful arthritic hip for several years, for which I have been taking anti-inflammatory drugs. However, this

treatment seems to have become less effective over the last few months. I expect I am too old for a hip replacement, so are there any alternative treatments?

Once drugs and physiotherapy fail to control the pain of a damaged or diseased hip joint, surgery may be the only viable alternative. You are not too old for a hip replacement operation; many people in their seventies, eighties and some even in their nineties have this type of surgery. Make an appointment to talk to your family doctor, who will probably refer you to an orthopaedic consultant for examination and assessment. You will need to have various tests to preclude any infection or other disease or condition which could complicate surgery or the use of an anaesthetic. It is important to be reasonably fit and well motivated before undergoing a hip replacement so that you have the best possible chance of regaining mobility and leading an active life afterwards. Your doctor and/or consultant will discuss with you the various factors to be considered, but surgery would not be precluded on the grounds of your age alone.

9.   *Having agreed to have a hip replacement operation, I am now very anxious about the prospect of having a general anaesthetic. Is there an alternative?*

It may be possible to have a spinal or epidural anaesthetic, both of which involve injection of the anaesthetic drug into the back to numb the nerves around the spinal cord. These anaesthetics are usually given in combination with a sedative which will put you to sleep during the operation itself.

If you are due to have a pre-operative assessment, ask the doctor or anaesthetist you see then about the possible anaesthetic options and explain the reasons for your anxiety about general anaesthesia. It may be that you are afraid of being given the anaesthetic through a face mask. If so, do mention this as very often face masks are only used when patients have already been put to sleep by the injection of a sedative.

Anaesthetics have improved dramatically over recent years and the risks associated with their use are now small. But whatever your specific worries, do voice them as medical staff should be able to reassure you and/or make sure you are given another type of anaesthesia if possible.

10.   *I had a total hip replacement about 11 years ago, at the age of 57, after which I led a very active life. Recently, however, I have started to have some pain in my hip and have been told that I need revision surgery. What does this entail and will it be as successful as my first operation, enabling me to carry on my life as normal afterwards?*

Revision surgery involves the removal of an existing replacement hip joint and the insertion of a new one. It is sometimes done in two separate operations, although usually in only one. First you will have several tests, including some to detect the presence of infection anywhere in your body. If you are found to have an infection, your existing hip joint will be removed and the infection treated over a period of a few weeks. During this time you will probably be able to walk with a walking aid, despite the fact that you have no hip joint. Once the infection has cleared, you will be re-admitted to hospital for your new hip joint to be inserted.

Alternatively, if there are no signs of infection, or possibly if there is only low-grade infection, your existing hip joint may be removed and the new implants inserted during a single operation. If your existing joint was cemented, the old cement will have to be chipped out before the new implants can be inserted. The operation can therefore take up to five hours or more and so is usually done under a general anaesthetic.

There is no reason why a revision hip joint should be any less successful than your existing one, although you may need to use walking sticks or crutches for a little longer than you did after your primary hip replacement. In addition, the hip may ache occasionally and may not last as long as the primary replacement.

11.   My wife is due to have a hemi-arthroplasty. What does this operation involve and how long will she be out of action after it?

A hemi-arthroplasty involves the removal and replacement of one side of the hip joint only. As it is usually done following fracture of the thigh bone, it is often the head of the thigh bone which is replaced. A prosthetic femoral head is inserted into cement in a channel made in the femur or is held in place by some form of cementless fixing.

Your wife will probably be in hospital for four or five days after her operation. Although she should be reasonably mobile when she leaves hospital, she will have to walk with sticks or crutches for at least a couple of months and will need help with household chores, shopping etc. during this time.

12.   My mother is 76, quite disabled by arthritis, and has to walk with two sticks. Although the pain in most of her joints has got a bit better recently, I think a hip replacement operation on her worst-affected leg would help her to get about more, although the consultant she saw does not agree. Why is the consultant reluctant to undertake surgery and can I ask for a second opinion for her?

You can, of course, ask for a second opinion, but it may be simpler to talk to your mother's consultant to discuss the reasons for his or her decision.

The main reasons for performing hip replacement surgery are to ease pain caused by damage or disease of the hip joint and to increase mobility. If your mother's pain can be controlled by drugs and if her activity is also restricted by arthritis in other joints, replacing her hip will not significantly alter her situation.

Hip replacement can dramatically improve the lives of people disabled by pain and immobility who wish to resume a reasonably active lifestyle, but it is a major operation and the reasons for doing it need to be carefully considered.

Do talk to your mother about what she wants to do, and

if having talked to her consultant you are still not satisfied - with the decision, ask her doctor for a referral for a second opinion.

13. I am 48 and have hip dysplasia which has recently caused me increasing problems. How long would a hip replacement last and would it be likely to need doing again during my lifetime?

It is not really possible to give an accurate estimate of how long a replacement hip would last, but probably the best guess would be up to 15 years, although it could be less than this, depending in part on your level of activity. However, having a hip replaced at your age would almost certainly mean that you would need revision surgery at some time in the future. Do talk to your family doctor, or ask for an appointment to be made for you with an orthopaedic consultant to discuss your options. If you are significantly disabled, the prospect of needing revision might be outweighed by the possible advantages to be gained from improving your lifestyle now.

14. I had a hip replaced a couple of years ago and now need another, unrelated operation. Should I tell the surgeon about my replacement hip?

Whenever you have any type of operation, you should mention any serious illness or surgery you have had in the past. It is particularly important in your case so that care can be taken to avoid dislocating your hip when you are under anaesthetic. You may need to have a course of antibiotics as a replacement hip must be protected from the risk of infection, which can increase with any form of surgery.

Case histories

The case histories which follow are not intended to make any specific points. They have been chosen at random as examples of the experiences of different men and women and are included simply to illustrate the reality of having hip replacement surgery for these people.

CASE 1

Marianne is 62. Two years ago, while staying in Australia, she woke up one morning with a severe, sharp pain in her left leg, from her waist to her foot. She thought it was sciatica or a pulled muscle and that it would go away. But after a couple of weeks of limping and constant pain, she went to see a doctor, whose diagnosis of a trapped nerve seemed to be supported by the lack of any X-ray evidence of abnormality. Over the next two to three months, the pain worsened and Marianne eventually went to a rheumatologist friend for advice. Further X-rays showed that the head of Marianne's thigh bone was rubbing against the socket in her pelvic bone and she was referred to an orthopaedic consultant and put on a waiting list for hip replacement surgery.

Before Marianne could have her operation, her plans changed and she returned to England, where she took her Australian X-rays to another orthopaedic surgeon. More X-rays were taken in London and she was given a full-body bone scan, but the surgeon was unable to detect any evidence of damage to the hip joint. He gave Marianne a steroid injection into her hip to try to ease the pain, but it had little effect. In desperation, she saw an orthopaedic consultant privately who confirmed that she did, indeed, need a total hip replacement. However, he agreed that the sudden onset of pain she had experienced was very unusual in cases of damage to the hip joint and that she could also have a trapped nerve.

Some 11 years previously, Marianne had undergone heart surgery in which her aortic valve had been replaced with one from a pig. She was therefore also assessed by a cardiac specialist and given a course of antibiotics. Because of her heart problem, she was unable to have warfarin or any other blood-thinning drugs and, following her hip replacement, she developed a deep vein thrombosis, which resolved before she was discharged from hospital after 10 days.

Marianne contacted the Department of Social Services from the private hospital she was in to ask for a raised toilet seat to use at home. Although she was told it would be waiting for her when she was discharged, it was another two weeks before it arrived, during which time she had to stand up to use the toilet. However, once the seat was delivered, she found the help she received from the DSS extremely good. A physiotherapist visited her at home until she was confident about using her hip.

Marianne is a very active person who travels regularly and she found the immobility in the months following her operation difficult to cope with. For the first three months, for example, she was unable to get on and off buses. She was also unprepared for the pain she suffered post-operatively, which continued for several months. She took painkillers regularly for the first three months, and two or three times a week for a further three months. It was almost a full year before she began to feel the real benefits of the operation and all her pain had gone (apart from an ache which develops when she becomes tired or walks too much). She lost a stone in weight after her hip operation, mostly, she feels, through anxiety. She remains indignant

at having been told by well-meaning friends that hip replacement surgery 'is like having a tooth pulled'!

CASE 2

Gordon is 58. About 11 years ago his knees became painful and
he started to have trouble rising from chairs. He saw a specialist,
had some X-rays taken and was told there were fragments of bone
in his knees. He took tablets for several months, with little effect.

Gordon then saw another orthopaedic consultant and had
several tests and examinations which revealed that the pain in
his knees was actually referred pain from his hips, particularly
the right one. His right hip was replaced about nine years ago.
Five years later, his left hip was also replaced, but this time the
wound failed to heal and over a period of six months was twice
re-opened surgically. Gordon was then advised that he would
need revision surgery. He had an operation to remove the components from his left hip, spent six weeks in hospital with his
leg in traction, and a further three months at home without a
hip joint. Although he was told that he could walk during this
period, he found it difficult and unpleasant to do so and was
thus more or less sedentary until he returned to hospital for the
new hip joint to be implanted. The operation was successful and
this time the wound healed satisfactorily.

Gordon was finally able to return to work, where he drives a
lorry and carries heavy bags of flour. His left leg aches a little if
he overdoes things, but the discomfort soon eases after half an
hour's rest. He has a check-up each year and is very pleased with
the final results of his operations.

Gordon's only 'problem' now is that, despite having a letter
(in English) from the hospital to explain that he has metal prostheses in his hips, he is regularly stopped and searched at foreign airports on his holidays abroad when the alarm sounds as
he passes through the metal detector.

CASE 3

Brian is 51. He was only 38 when he first developed pain, in his left and then in his right hip. Despite several tests, including a full-body scan, it was some time before the cause was discovered. Brian underwent an osteotomy on each hip in an attempt to transfer the force exerted during walking away from the damaged areas of his thigh bones. But the pain continued, and he was only able to walk with crutches.

Some three years after his hip problems first started, Brian was told by his consultant that both his hip joints needed to be replaced. He was one of the first people in Britain to be given cementless prostheses. The first operation was successful, although he did have some discomfort for a few weeks afterwards due to bruising of the sciatic nerve. About eight months later, Brian had another operation to replace the hip joint in his other leg.

Some 10 years later, Brian occasionally has pain in his left hip which lasts for three to four days, during which time he uses a walking stick. He has an annual check-up and a couple of years ago was added to the waiting list for revision surgery for his left hip. However, the minor problems apparent then seemed to resolve and the following year his name was removed from the list.

Before his operations, and only in his late thirties, Brian was almost crippled by pain and disability. He had had to give up his job, was unable to walk up and down stairs, and could not put on his own shoes or socks. His life has changed dramatically since then and, although he has been unable to return to work, he is virtually pain free and can once again lead a normal life.

CASE 4

Irene is 75. Some 15 years ago, she began to have a slight ache in her right hip and eventually went to see her doctor, who arranged for an X-ray to be taken. The X-ray showed signs of the early stages of arthritis and Irene was given anti-inflammatory tablets which she continued to take – on a repeat prescription – for several years. Her arthritis gradually progressed until the tablets became ineffective, by which time she had pain in both her hips and severely restricted mobility.

Irene returned to her doctor about three years ago and an appointment was made for X-rays to be taken of both her hips. These revealed significant destruction and very little movement of the hip joints, and a couple of months later Irene was admitted to hospital for surgery to replace her right hip joint with cemented implants. Her left hip was replaced about four months later, the implants this time being fixed with screws.

By the time she was admitted to hospital for her second operation, Irene was reasonably mobile and walking with two sticks. She used crutches until her second hip joint had stabilised, but now only takes a walking stick to support her on particularly long walks.

Irene realised the importance of exercising and following all the instructions she had been given by hospital staff after her operations, and the effort she put into her rehabilitation paid off. She is very pleased with the success of her operations and would advise anyone contemplating hip replacement surgery to go ahead.

CASE 5

Brief details of Carla's unusual case history have been included as an example of what it may be possible to achieve with perseverance.

Carla is 40. When she was 17, she was involved in a serious road accident, suffering multiple injuries, including fracturing both her femurs and dislocating her right hip joint. She underwent a series of operations, during one of which the fractures were mended and her right hip joint was put back in place.

Seven years later, after a year of increasing pain and reduced mobility, Carla had another operation to resurface the head of the femur and replace her right hip with cemented prostheses. She suffered an allergic reaction to the anaesthetic used during this operation, and all her subsequent operations were carried out using epidural anaesthesia and a sedative.

Unfortunately, her replaced hip failed and a year later she underwent revision surgery in which Charnley prostheses were inserted. The femoral component was replaced again the following year as it had come loose on several occasions. Four years later, Carla underwent plastic surgery to her right hip following breakdown of the wound, possibly as a result of an allergic reaction. The next year she had her fourth total hip replacement, this time using uncemented fixation, after which she suffered a deep vein thrombosis and two pulmonary emboli.

Carla had her fifth total hip replacement a year later – again with uncemented fixation – but the hip joint failed to stabilise and after a few months the femur snapped. After two months in bed she could only walk with crutches. Later that same year, her right hip was replaced for the sixth time. Although the operation was successful, the hip joint was dislocated during a post-operative X-ray and Carla had to wear a hip brace for some time. For the past year, she has remained reasonably mobile and pain free.

Medical terms

Abduction   Moving away from the midline of the body.

Abduction pillow   A triangular cushion which is often placed between the legs following hip replacement surgery to keep them in the correct position (abducted) until a patient who has been anaesthetised is able to control their movements again.

Abscess   A collection of pus secondary to localised infection. Pus forms as a result of inflammation and is a fluid containing dead cells, fragments of tissue and sometimes bacteria.

Acetabular component   An artificial implant inserted to replace the acetabulum on the pelvis and to articulate with the head of the thigh bone.

Acetabulum   The cup-shaped socket on the outer surface of the pelvic bone into which the head of the thigh bone fits.

Adduction   Moving towards the midline of the body.

Adductor muscle   A muscle which draws a part, such as the leg, towards the central axis of the body.

Allergy   An abnormal reaction to a substance. An allergic reaction can be mild, causing an itchy rash, or severe, leading to fainting, vomiting, loss of consciousness or death.

Allograft   A graft between two individuals of the same species.

Alloy A mixture of two or more metals.

Anaesthesia   The absence of sensation.

Anaesthetic   A drug which causes loss of sensation in part or all of the body.

Anaesthetist   A doctor trained in the administration of anaesthetics.

Analgesic   A drug which blocks the sensation of pain; a painkiller.

Ankylosing spondylitis   A degenerative or non-inflammatory disease of the spine which causes damage to the joints between the vertebrae, leading to immobility of the affected parts of the vertebral column. It may also affect the hips and other large joints.

Antibiotic   A substance which kills bacteria or prevents them replicating.

Anticoagulant   A substance which thins the blood and prevents it from clotting.

Anti-embolism stockings   Stockings sometimes worn during an operation and during any period of immobilisation post-operatively. The stockings assist the circulation of blood in the legs and help to prevent blood clots forming.

Anti-emetic   A drug which helps to reduce feelings of sickness.

Arthritis   Inflammation of a joint. There are various types of arthritis, such as osteoarthritis and rheumatoid arthritis, the causes of which are not always known.

Arthropathy   Any disease affecting a joint.

Arthroplasty   Surgical reconstruction of a joint, with or without an implant.

Articular cartilage   Cartilage which covers the articulating surfaces of a synovial joint, such as the hip joint.

Aseptic loosening   Loosening of an artificial component in a replacement joint which is not due to infection.

Aspiration   The withdrawal of fluid or gas from a body cavity using suction.

Atrophy   Wasting away due to lack of nourishment or use.

Autograft   A graft of skin or other tissue taken from one part of the body to correct a defect in another part of the same individual.

Ball-and-socket joint   A joint formed by the round part of a bone fitting into a cup-shaped cavity in another bone, e.g. the hip joint.

Biological fixation   A technique involving coating a prosthesis with a porous layer, such as cobalt chrome beads or titanium mesh, to induce ingrowth of bone into it.

Biomechanics   The science of forces acting on an organism or on part of an organism.

Biopsy   The surgical removal of a piece of tissue from a living body for examination under a microscope to assist or confirm a diagnosis.

Bone stock   The quality of bone.

Bone bank   A place where bone is stored in very cold freezers for use in grafting.

Cannula   A very fine tube or needle. Fluids can be introduced into or removed from the body through an intravenous cannula which has been inserted into a vein, usually in the back of the hand. Anaesthetic drugs are administered through an intravenous catheter during an operation. Cannulas are usually made of plastic, but used to be metal or glass.

Cartilage   A specialised body tissue which is firm but flexible, such as that covering the articulating surfaces of bone in a synovial joint.

Catheter   A thin tube used to withdraw fluid from or introduce it into the body.

Cauterise   To burn a part with heat or some other agent. During surgery, the severed ends of small blood vessels are sealed with the tip of an instrument heated by an electric current to stop them bleeding.

Cement-fixed prosthesis   An artificial implant which is fixed in place using cement.

Cementless prosthesis   An artificial implant which is fixed in place without the use of cement.

Ceramic   A substance produced by heating clay and minerals to a high temperature to give it strength and make it hard. It may be used as an articular surface or as a bioactive coating in joint implants.

Cobalt chrome   An alloy of the hard metals cobalt and chrome which is tough and malleable.

Complication   A condition which occurs as the result of another disease or condition. It may also be an unwanted side-effect of treatment.

Component   An artificial part used to replace a body part; a prosthesis or implant.

Computer tomography (CT)   A scan which takes X-rays through 'slices' of the body. The images are interpreted by a computer to build up a three-dimensional picture.

Congenital   Present from birth.

Congenital hip dysplasia   Abnormal development of the hip joint which is present from birth.

Connective tissue   Fibrous tissue which connects and supports organs within the body.

Consent form   A form which patients must sign before surgery to confirm that they understand what is involved in their operation and give their consent for it to take place. Signing the form also gives consent for the use of anaesthetic drugs and any other procedures which doctors feel to be necessary during surgery.

Consultant   An experienced and fully trained doctor who specialises in a particular type of medicine.

Contracture   Deformity caused by shortening of muscle.

Cross-match   Matching of the blood of a potential recipient with that from a donor to ensure that blood of the same group is given by transfusion, for example after an operation involving significant blood loss.

Day-case surgery   Surgery for which a patient is in hospital for one day only, with no overnight stay.

Deep vein thrombosis (DVT)   A blood clot in a deep vein, often in the lower leg or pelvis.

Degenerative disease   Any disease involving the breaking down of an organ or tissue, thus affecting its form and/or function.

Diagnosis   The identification of a disease based on its symptoms and signs.

Diathermy   A method of generating heat by means of a high-frequency electric current. It is used in surgery to destroy diseased tissue or to stop bleeding from damaged blood vessels.

Direct closure   The drawing together of the edges of a wound with stitches.

Discharge letter   A letter given to patients leaving hospital (or sent directly from the hospital) to deliver to their family doctor. It gives details of the treatment they have received and any follow-up required.

Dislocation   Complete displacement of one bone in relation to another at a joint.

Drain   Often a tube, which may be attached to a bag or bottle, which is inserted into a wound to drain away excess blood and fluid.

Drip/Intravenous infusion   A tube used to administer fluid to replace that lost from the body after an operation or injury. One end is inserted into a vein in an arm and the other end is attached to a bottle or bag containing a specially balanced saline or sugar solution.

Dura (mater)   The tough outer membrane which surrounds the brain and spinal cord in a protective sheath.

Electrocardiogram (ECG)   The activity of the heart recorded as a series of electrical wave patterns.

Electrocautery   The application of the electrically heated tip of an instrument to the ends of blood vessels to stop them bleeding.

Embolus (plural: **emboli**)   A piece of a blood clot (or air bubble) which has broken away and can pass through the blood vessels. If it lodges in a vital organ, such as the lung, it can have fatal consequences.

Epidural anaesthetic   An anaesthetic drug which is injected outside the dura into the space around the nerves in the back. It causes numbness in the legs and groin which lasts for three to five hours. Epidurals are used for pain relief and/or to produce loss of sensation during surgery to the legs or lower body.

Erythema   Redness due to increased blood flow.

Excision   Removal by cutting.

Excision arthroplasty   The surgical removal of a joint.

Extension   Straightening, for example of a bent limb.

External rotation   Rotation, for example of a limb, away from the body.

Femoral component   An artificial implant inserted to replace part of the thigh bone.

Femur   The thigh bone.

Fibrosis   The development of excessive fibrous tissue.

Fixed Price Care   The system used by some private hospitals whereby a fixed price is quoted for a particular type of operation and some of the hospitalisation costs associated with it.

Flexion   The bending of a joint so that the two parts connected by it come together.

Flexion contracture   Shortening of muscle which causes the bones on either side of a joint to come into close contact with each other.

Foreign body reaction   The body's reaction to the presence of some substance which is not usually found within it. Large inflammatory cells accumulate around the foreign material in an attempt to seal it off and isolate it.

Fracture   A break, particularly of a bone.

Gait   Way of walking.

General anaesthetic   A drug which induces loss of consciousness and abolishes the sensation of pain in all parts of the body.

Gluteus muscle   One of the three muscles of the buttocks which runs from the pelvic bone to the head of the femur.

Graft   A piece of tissue removed from one site and placed at another to repair a defect resulting from an operation, accident or disease. The tissue can be taken from the same or another individual.

Haematoma   A blood-filled swelling. A haematoma can form in a wound after an operation if blood continues to leak from a blood vessel. If the blood spreads in the tissues, it appears as a bruise.

Haemoglobin   An iron-containing pigment in red blood cells which carries oxygen molecules around the body.

Haemophilia   An inherited disease, transmitted by women but normally affecting only men, in which the mechanism of blood clotting is faulty, leading to uncontrolled bleeding when a blood vessel is severed.

Haemorrhage   Bleeding.

Hemi-arthroplasty   The replacement of one half of a joint with an artificial implant.

Heparin   A substance which occurs naturally in the body and which helps to prevent the blood clotting. It may be given by injection before and after surgery to people who are at particular risk of developing blood clots.

Heterotopic bone formation   The development of bone at a site at which it would not normally occur.

Histological examination   The microscopic examination of a sample of tissue which has been taken from the body by biopsy.

Hybrid replacement   Total hip replacement involving the insertion of a cementless acetabular prosthesis and a cement-fixed femoral prosthesis. This operation seems to be successful, although no long-term results are as yet available.

Hydroxyapatite   A chemical compound, containing calcium phosphate, from which bone salts are derived.

Hypothermia   A condition in which the temperature of the body is abnormally low.

Iliacus muscle   A muscle which runs along the inner aspect of the pelvis down to the femur.

Ilium   The upper part of the pelvis on which the acetabulum is situated.

Incision   A cut or wound made by a sharp instrument, such as during an operation.

Incontinence   Lack of voluntary control over the discharge of urine or faeces.

Induction agent   A drug used in anaesthesia to bring on loss of consciousness.

Inhalational anaesthetic   An anaesthetic given as a mixture of gases which is inhaled, usually to maintain anaesthesia.

Inflammation   The response of a tissue to injury or infection which involves the rush of blood and white blood cells to the affected part, causing redness, swelling and pain.

Internal rotation   Rotation, for example of a limb, towards the central axis of the body.

Interpositional arthroplasty   An operation to interpose a material between the ends of bones or the surfaces of a joint to keep them apart.

Intravenous anaesthetic   A general anaesthetic drug which is injected into a vein via a cannula, usually in the back of the hand.

Intra-operative   Occurring during an operation.

Ischium   The bone forming the lower, posterior part of the pelvis.

Joint   The junction of two or more bones which enables them to move relative to each other.

Joint cavity   The space between the bones of a joint which is filled with synovial fluid; synovial cavity.

Ligament   A tough, flexible strand of fibrous tissue which connects bones and contributes towards the stability of joints.

Local anaesthetic   An anaesthetic which numbs the area of the body around which it is injected.

Local injection   An injection of a substance which remains confined to one area and is not distributed throughout the body.

Lymph   A pale-coloured fluid which flows within the lymphatic vessels of the body and is eventually returned to the blood. It contains disease-fighting cells, the lymphocytes.

Lymphocyte   A type of white blood cell involved in fighting disease in the body.

Lymphoedema   A condition in which the lymphatic drainage of part of the body is impaired, causing swelling, tightness of the skin and pain as the lymph collects.

Magnetic resonance imaging (MRI)   The use of a large magnet to produce a magnetic field in individual cells of the body. An energy field is applied which affects the alignment of atoms within the cells and causes them to emit a signal which is detected by a computer and interpreted as an image of the body. The procedure is very useful for visualising soft tissues which are not seen on routine X-rays.

Maintenance agent   A drug used during an operation to maintain the state of general anaesthesia.

Metastatic infection   Infection which has spread from a primary site to another part of the body, either directly or via the blood or lymphatic vessels.

Nasogastric tube   A tube inserted via a nostril after some operations to drain the stomach and prevent vomiting. A smaller version is sometimes used to introduce a specially balanced fluid into the stomach to feed patients who are unable to eat.

National Health Service (NHS)   The system of medical care, set up in Britain in 1948, under which medical treatment is mostly funded by taxation.

Nausea   A feeling of sickness.

Necrosis   Death of tissue.

Nerve palsy   Loss of function in some part of the body due to damage to its nerves.

Neuroma   A swelling of nerve cells and nerve fibres.

Neuropathy   A condition involving the destruction or degeneration of the tissue of the central or peripheral nerves, caused by drugs or metabolic or vascular disturbance.

Nil by mouth   A term used to mean that no food or drink should be swallowed in the hours before an operation.

Nodule   A small swelling of cells.

Non-steroidal anti-inflammatory drug (NSAID)   A drug which suppresses inflammation but which is not a steroid, for example indomethacin and ibuprofen.

Obesity   An excessive amount of fat in the body. This term is non-specific and is being replaced by a figure calculated from height and weight measurements, known as the **body mass index**.

Occupational therapist   Someone trained to assist people in their recovery from disease, injury or surgery by means of mental or physical activity.

One-stage revision   The removal of the components of a hip replacement and insertion of new components during a single operation.

Orthopaedic surgery   Surgery which deals with abnormalities, diseases and injury to the locomotor system, i.e. any part of the body involved in movement.

Osseo-integration   The process of growth of bone into another substance.

Ossification   The formation of bone.

Osteoarthritis   Inflammation of a joint, particularly of the hip, spine and hands, which causes it to degenerate. It is often age related but may result from severe or repeated injury or from abnormal alignment. Osteoarthritis of the knee may be a result of obesity.

Osteolysis   The breaking down and absorption of bone or the loss of calcium from it.

Osteophyte   Outgrowth of bone at the edge of a joint.

Osteoporosis   An increase in the porosity of bone due to loss of minerals from it. It may occur with increasing age, particularly in post-menopausal women, and makes the bones brittle and prone to fracture.

Osteotome   A chisel-like surgical instrument used to cut a bone.

Osteotomy   An operation which involves cutting through bone.

It may be done to realign bones and to redistribute the load through the adjacent joint.

Osteotomy arthroplasty An operation involving cutting through a bone.

Pectineus muscle A small muscle in the groin between the pubis of the pelvis and the femur which adducts and flexes the hip joint.

Pelvis The basin-shaped ring of bone at the lower end of the trunk of the body which protects the pelvic organs and is formed by the fusion of three component bones.

Physiotherapy The use of physical measures to build muscle strength, correct deformity and restore function after disease, injury or surgery.

Polyethylene A synthetic resin which is tough and flexible.

Polymer A compound formed from repeated units of one or more compounds.

Polymethylmethacrylate A chemical constituent of bone cement.

Post-operative Following an operation.

Pre-clerking admission procedure/Pre-operative assessment A procedure used in some hospitals whereby patients attend an appointment a few days or weeks before an operation for any necessary pre-operative tests, such as blood tests and ECGs, the results of which are thus available when the patient is admitted for surgery.

Pre-medication ('Pre-med.') A drug which is given before another drug, for example one given an hour or two before an operation to relax the patient before anaesthesia is started.

Pre-operative Before an operation.

Primary hip replacement An operation to replace the bones of the hip joint for the first time.

Prognosis An opinion about the probable course and final outcome of a disease which is made when all the known facts are considered.

Prophylactic Something used to prevent a disease or condition developing.

Prosthesis An artificial part.

Psoas muscle A muscle extending from the side of the vertebral column to the upper part of the thigh bone which flexes the hip joint.

Pubis The front part of the hip bone (pelvis).

Pulmonary embolism A blood clot or air bubble which blocks the blood vessels in the lung.

Pyrexia A fever.

Reamer A small surgical instrument used to make or enlarge a cavity in bone, for example to insert a femoral or acetabular component during a hip replacement operation.

Recovery room A ward near the operating theatre to which patients are taken after surgery so that they can be closely watched while they recover from a general anaesthetic.

Rectus femoris muscle The muscle which runs between the front part of the ilium of the pelvis and the knee cap and which plays a minor role in flexing the hip.

Referred pain Pain felt in one part of the body which arises as a result of damage or disease in another part.

Regional anaesthesia Anaesthesia of a specific area of the body.

Rehabilitation Training to restore the use of a part of the body which has been lost or reduced following injury, disease or surgery.

Revision surgery Surgery which is repeated due to the failure of an earlier operation.

Rheumatoid arthritis Inflammation, typically of multiple joints, causing pain, weakness and eventually deformity and loss of function. Its causes are unknown.

Sacrum The bone at the back of the pelvis which is formed by fusion of five sacral vertebrae.

Sepsis Infection caused by pus-producing bacteria.

Septicaemia Severe infection caused by large numbers of bacteria in the blood which multiply and spread; blood poisoning.

Seroma A collection of clear fluid, such as lymph, which may develop following an operation. If persistent, the fluid can be drawn off with a needle.

Shaft (of bone) The long, cylindrical part of a bone.

Side-effect An effect other than that desired which results from the use of a drug or other form of treatment.

Sign Something a doctor looks for as an indication of disease, such as a lesion or swelling.

Skin graft A piece of skin taken from one site on the body to replace that which has been lost because of injury or surgery at another site.

Spinal anaesthetic An anaesthetic which is injected between the vertebrae of the spine into the space around the nerves in the back. It causes numbness in the legs and groin which lasts for three to five hours.

Stasis The slowing down or cessation of flow of a fluid. Blood stasis causes pooling of blood within a blood vessel.

Steroid One of a group of naturally occurring substances in the body which includes some hormones.

Subluxation Incomplete dislocation of a joint.

Suture A surgical stitch or row of stitches.

Symphysis pubis The point at which the pubic bones unite.

Symptom Something experienced by a patient which indicates a disturbance of normal body function, for example pain or nausea.

Synovial fluid The fluid secreted by the synovial membrane and present in the space between the bones of a joint which nourishes and lubricates the ends of the bones.

Synovial joint A mobile joint, the bones of which are separated by synovial fluid.

Synovitis Inflammation of the synovial membrane of a joint. It is usually accompanied by the collection of synovial fluid within the joint cavity, and thus by swelling.

Synovium   The membrane around a joint cavity which secretes synovial fluid.

Tensor fascia lata   A muscle which runs from the ilium of the pelvis to the femur and which stretches the hip joint.

Thrombo-embolic deterrent stockings (TEDS)   *See* Anti-embolism stockings.

Thromboplastin   A substance which is released into the bloodstream when blood is shed and which plays a role in the formation of a blood clot.

Thrombosis   The coagulation of blood within a vein or artery which produces a blood clot.

Thrombus   A blood clot which remains within the blood vessel in which it forms.

Titanium   A metal present in certain ores.

Titanium alloy   A combination of the metal titanium with iron or copper.

Trochanter   One of the two bony prominences at the upper end of the thigh bone.

Two-stage revision   Revision surgery done in two separate operations. During the first, the components of hip replacement are removed, and during the second, often six weeks or more later, the bone is reconstructed and the new components are inserted. Any infection or other complication is treated during the period between the two operations.

Ulcer   A lesion of the skin in which the surface layers have been destroyed, exposing the deeper tissues.

Urinalysis   The analysis of urine to detect the presence of certain chemicals and/or of bacteria.

Urinary retention   Retention of urine in the bladder caused by obstruction to its flow or weakness of the muscles of the bladder wall.

Warfarin   An anticoagulant which may be used to treat thrombosis by thinning the blood and helping to dissolve the blood clot.

Wear debris   Small particles which are rubbed off the articulating surfaces of prostheses as a result of the friction between them. The particles can set up an inflammatory reaction, causing breakdown and absorption of the surrounding bone, and eventually loosening of the prostheses themselves.

Xenograft   A graft between a donor and a recipient of a different species.

X-ray   A type of electromagnetic radiation of short wavelength which is able to pass through opaque bodies. It can be used in diagnosis, by allowing the visualisation of internal structures and organs of the body, or in higher doses as therapy to destroy malignant cells.

Useful addresses

There are various organisations in most countries throughout the world which provide advice, information and, in some cases, practical support. A few of those in the UK are listed here, but the addresses of arthritis societies or foundations can be found in your telephone directory. Your hospital or health department should also be able to supply details of any other useful organisations in your area.

Disabled Living Centres/Independent Living Centres

There are centres throughout the UK, the addresses of which can be obtained from a telephone directory or from the Disabled Living Foundation (see below). They provide free and independent advice about the assistance available, both practical and financial, and at many you can see and try out various aids before deciding whether to buy. Many of the staff are physiotherapists or occupational therapists.

The Disabled Living Foundation

380–384 Harrow Road
London W9 2HU
Telephone: 0171 289 6111

The Disabled Living Foundation provides advice on aids and appliances for the home.

Mobility Advice and Vehicle Information Service
Department of Transport
TRL
Crowthorne
Berkshire RG45 6AU
Telephone: 01344 770456

This service was set up by the Department of Transport and provides assessment of driving ability and practical advice on possible car adaptations for both drivers and passengers with disability. Contact the service at Crowthorne for the addresses of other centres around the country.

The Arthritis and Rheumatism Council
Copeman House
St Mary's Court
St Mary's Gate
Chesterfield
Derbyshire S41 7TD
Telephone: 01246 558033

This is a charitable organisation which funds research projects into rheumatic diseases and produces a range of leaflets giving explanations and practical advice.

Arthritis Care
18 Stephenson Way
London NW1 2HD
Telephone: 0171 916 1500 (open 10 a.m. to 4 p.m., Monday to Friday)
Helpline: Freephone 0800 289170 (open 12 a.m. to 4 p.m., Monday to Friday)

Free confidential advice and information are available, by letter or phone, from a counselling team.

The Royal Association for Disability & Rehabilitation

25 Mortimer Street
London W1N 8AB
Telephone: 0171 250 3222

Information and advice can be obtained from this national organisation, including details of national and local groups and of the entitlement to various social services etc. of those with particular disabilities.

Department of Social Services

There may be community occupational therapists based at your local Department of Social Services who can give you advice and home assessment, although there may be some delay before an appointment can be made for you. The address and phone number of your local DSS will be in your telephone directory.

How to complain

If you are unhappy about anything that has occurred – or, indeed, that has not occurred – during your stay in hospital, there are several possible paths to follow if you want to make a complaint.

However, before you set the complaints machinery in motion, you should give careful thought to what is involved. Once a formal complaint has been made against a doctor and the complaints procedure has begun, there is little chance of stopping it.

If you think you have a genuine grievance, do try to talk to the person concerned, explaining as clearly and unemotionally as possible what it is that you feel has gone wrong. If you do not feel able to discuss things directly, you can always present your case in a letter.

The vast majority of doctors – family doctors and those who work in hospitals – are dedicated, conscientious and hard working. They really do have their patients' best interests at heart, and many work very long hours each week, night and day. A complaint against a doctor is usually a devastating blow, which can cause considerable stress. Of course, if something has gone wrong during your medical treatment, you may also have suffered stress and unhappiness, but before you make an official complaint, do consider whether your doctor's actions have really warranted what many would see as a 'kick in the teeth'.

The best approach is to make a polite and reasoned enquiry to the person concerned. However angry or irritated you may feel, a complaint made aggressively, however justified this may seem, is unlikely to achieve much.

The following brief sections explain how to make an official complaint in the UK. Leaflets and other information giving details of all the appropriate councils and complaints procedures and how they work can be obtained from your hospital or local health authority. If you have any problems with the offices mentioned below, information about what to do and who to go to for help is available from Citizens Advice Bureaus and Community Health Councils.

HOSPITAL STAFF

If your complaint concerns something that has happened during your stay in hospital and for some reason you are unable to approach the person directly concerned, you can talk to the ward sister or charge nurse, the hospital doctor on your ward, or the senior manager for the department or ward. Many complaints can be dealt with directly by one of these people, but if this is not possible, they will be able to refer you to the appropriate person.

THE GENERAL MANAGER

If you are intimidated by the thought of speaking to one of the people mentioned above, you can write to the hospital's General Manager, sometimes called the Director of Operations or Chief Executive. The General Manager has responsibility for the way the hospital is run.

The Government's Patients' Charter states that anyone making a complaint about an NHS service must receive a 'full and prompt written reply from the Chief Executive or General Manager'. You should therefore receive an immediate response to your letter, and your complaint should be fully investigated by a senior manager.

The hospital switchboard, or any medical or clerical staff at the hospital, should be able to give you the General Manager's name and office address. If you would prefer to do so, you can make an appointment to speak to him or her, rather than writing a letter.

Depending on how serious your complaint is, you should receive either a full report of the investigation into it or regular letters telling you what is happening until such a report can be made. Do make sure you keep copies of all letters you write and receive concerning your complaint.

DISTRICT HEALTH AUTHORITY

If the treatment you require is not available in your area, or the waiting list is very long, you can contact your local District Health Authority. The District Health Authority is able to deal with complaints concerning the provision of services, rather than with those resulting from something going wrong with your treatment. The District Health Authority can sometimes arrange for you to have treatment elsewhere where waiting lists are shorter, if this is what you want.

Your NHS authority should produce a leaflet to explain how it deals with complaints which will be available at your hospital or clinic. If you have any difficulty finding out who to contact, write to the General Manager of the hospital. Someone at the hospital will be able to tell you which health authority covers the area in which you live.

COMMUNITY HEALTH COUNCIL

Independent advice and assistance can be obtained from your local Community Health Council. Someone from the Community Health Council will be able to explain the complaints procedures to you, help you to write letters to the hospital, and also come with you to any meetings arranged between hospital representatives and yourself. Again, the address of the Community Health Council for your area can be obtained from a hospital or local telephone directory.

REGIONAL MEDICAL OFFICER

If your complaint concerns the standard of *clinical* treatment you received in hospital, and the paths you have already taken have not led to a satisfactory conclusion, you can take it to the Regional Medical Officer for your area.

FAMILY HEATLH SERVICES AUTHORITY

Family doctors are now encouraged to have their own 'in-house' complaints services, but a complaint about your family doctor which you have been unable to sort out by this means can be reported to the Family Health Services Authority. Such complaints should be made within 13 weeks of the incident occurring. Again, your local Community Health Council will be able to give you advice and help you make your complaint and write letters etc.

HEALTH SERVICE COMMISSIONER

If all else has failed, you can take your complaint to the Health Service Commissioner. The commissioner is independent of both the NHS and the government, being responsible to Parliament.

The Health Service Commissioner is able to deal with complaints made by individuals about the failure of a NHS authority to provide the service it should – a failure which has caused actual hardship or injustice. You must have taken your complaint up with your local health authority first, but if you have not received a satisfactory response within a reasonable time, write to the Health Service Commissioner enclosing copies of *all* the relevant letters and documents as well as giving details of the incident itself. The Health Commissioner is not able to investigate complaints about clinical treatment.

You must contact the Health Service Commissioner within *one* year of the incident occurring, unless there is some valid reason why you have been unable to do so.

There is a separate Health Service Commissioner for each country within the United Kingdom.

Health Service Commissioner for England
Church House
Great Smith Street
London SW1P 3BW
Telephone: 0171 276 2035

Health Service Commissioner for Scotland
Second Floor
11 Melville Crescent
Edinburgh EH3 7LU
Telephone: 0131 225 7465

Health Service Commissioner for Wales
4th Floor Pearl Assurance House
Greyfriars Road
Cardiff CF1 3AG
Telephone: 01222 394621

Office of the Northern Ireland Commissioner for Complaints
33 Wellington Place
Belfast BT1 6HN
Telephone: 01232 233821

TAKING LEGAL ACTION

The legal path is likely to be an expensive one, and should be a last resort rather than a starting point.

In theory, everyone has a right to take legal action. However, unless you have very little money and are entitled to Legal Aid, or a great deal of money, you are unlikely to be able to afford this costly process. The outcome of legal action can never be assured, and the possible cost if you lose your case should be borne in mind.

If you do think you have grounds for compensation for injury caused to you as a result of negligence, advice can be sought from:

The Association for the Victims of Medical Accidents (AVMA)
1 London Road
Forest Hill
London SE23 3TP
Telephone: 0181 291 2793.

Someone from the AVMA will be able to give you free and confidential legal advice about whether or not you have a case worth pursuing. They will also be able to recommend solicitors with training in medical law who may be prepared to represent you.

SUMMARY

Do tell nursing or other medical staff if you are not happy about *any* aspect of your care in hospital. They may be able to deal with your complaint immediately. But do remember, if the matter is a serious one, or if you are not satisfied with the response you receive, you are entitled to pursue it through all the levels that exist to deal with such problems.

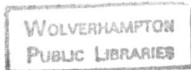

Index